This is one of the easiest-to-follow, easiest-to-apply guides to foot care ever produced, and it deserves a comfortable, dry, and cozy spot in every runner's travel bag, triathlete's fanny pack, and backpacker's rucksack.

—**Richard Benyo, author of Death Valley 300 and
Making the Marathon Your Event, and
editor of Marathon & Beyond magazine**

Fixing Your Feet is the definitive guide to foot care. I read this book while preparing for my 7400-mile Calendar Triple Crown hike. Solo most of the time for a year on the trail, I needed to be my own foot-care expert, and this book taught me what I needed to know.

—**Brian Robinson, the first person to hike the Appalachian,
the Continental Divide, and the Pacific Crest trails
in a calendar year**

This is a book for people who want common sense treatments for foot problems, not classroom or clinic theories of little value. I am providing copies for my patients and making this required reading at my sports-injury lectures.

—**David Hannaford, DPM, sports podiatrist to many
Olympians, ultramarathoners, adventure racers, and
other endurance athletes**

Fixing Your Feet is a must for any long or ultra-distance runner, hiker, triathlete, or adventure racer. Your chances of successful training and racing will be greatly improved after having read this book.

—**Don D Mann, race director for The Beast of the East,
The Mega Dose, The Odyssey Double and Triple Iron,
The Expedition British Virgin Island Adventure Race,
and Race to the Pole**

Fixing Your Feet is for those of us who hike, backpack, run, or do any active outdoor sport that pounds our feet. It teaches that conquering blisters (and other foot ailments) is a very personal affair. What works for one person, doesn't work for another. And what works for you today may cease to work for you in the future.

—**Sue Freeman, Footprint Press and hiker**

Should an ultrarunner own *Fixing Your Feet*? Should a preacher own a Bible? If you don't have it, get it. Blisters are not mandatory.

—Will Brown, ultrarunner

The first ultra I did was the Ohlone Wilderness 50K Trail Run, and my feet were so blistered by the 20-mile mark that I almost dropped. After reading *Fixing Your Feet,* things have changed for the better. I ran the Skyline 50K with no foot problems and hiked to summit of Mt. Whitney with no complications. Thanks for the good advice. Your book will remain in my library for years to come.

—Brett Lehigh, ultrarunner

Fixing Your Feet is an often-referred-to reference on my bookshelf for me, my wife, my daughter (for cramped toes from wearing high heels for a beauty pageant!) and boys in soccer, basketball, and track. It contains a great collection of strategies and advice for just about anything that can go wrong with your feet. Not one thing will help everyone's foot problem, and John recognizes this, giving you multiple strategies to try out.

—Greg "Strider" Hummel, thru-hiker

The most comprehensive, highly readable (even enjoyable) book on foot care I have seen. A "must have" resource book for every athlete's library!

—Pat Wellington, ultrarunner

I'm not an athlete, just a "40-something" struggling to keep fit. I'm hoping to be able to continue doing my daily moderate 3-mile dirt road up-and-down loop walk for many years to come. This year it hit me: I have to take care of my feet—proactively—or I may not be able to continue walking well into my senior years. With this book, I'm confident I can deal with some emerging problems (calluses, bunions, etc.) and prevent others. The detailed information on boots and socks was especially helpful. Obviously, this book is great for athletes, for dabblers like me, and I would imagine for anyone who spends a lot of time on the job on his/her feet.

—Populore, Morgantown, West Virginia

Fixing Your Feet is a "must read" for any thru-hiker! I have learned much more in reading in one afternoon than in 25 years of hiking.

—Monte Dodge, thru-hiker

FIXING YOUR
Feet
prevention and treatments
for athletes

John Vonhof

Third Edition

 WILDERNESS PRESS · BERKELEY, CA

Fixing Your Feet: Prevention and Treatments for Athletes

1st EDITION 1997
2nd EDITION 2000
3rd EDITION May 2004

Copyright © 1997, 2000, 2004 by John Vonhof

Front cover photo copyright © 2004 by Wilderness Press
Back cover illustration copyright © 1997, 2000, 2004 by Adam Caldwell
Interior photos, except where noted, by John Vonhof
Interior illustrations by John Vonhof
Cover design and front cover photo: Andreas Schueller
Book design and layout: Emily Douglas
Book editor: Kate Hoffman

ISBN 0-89997-354-X
UPC 7-19609-97354-6

Manufactured in the United States of America

Published by: **Wilderness Press**
1200 5th Street
Berkeley, CA 94710
(800) 443-7227; FAX (510) 558-1696
info@wildernesspress.com
www.wildernesspress.com

Visit our website for a complete listing of our books and for ordering information.

Many of the designations used by manufacturers and sellers to distinguish their products are claimed as trademarks. Where those designations appear in this book and the author is aware of a trademark claim, they are identified by initial capital letters. These products are listed in alphabetical order for the sake of simplicity. The order does not imply one product is more helpful or less helpful than another.

SAFETY NOTICE: Although Wilderness Press and the author have made every attempt to ensure that the information in this book is accurate at press time, they are not responsible for any loss, damage, injury, or inconvenience that may occur as a result of using this book. The information contained here is no substitute for professional advice or training. Readers are encouraged to seek medical help whenever possible.

Foreword

I ran my first ultramarathon at age 15, and during it I became painfully aware that an athlete's feet are one of the most important parts of the body. Shortly after that first ultra, I was competing at the World Ride and Tie Championships with Ken "Cowman" Shirk. Before the race, while rinsing his feet, he leaned over and said, "Take good care of your feet and they will take you wherever you want to go." Over the next 23 years, as I participated in 236 ultramarathons, trail runs, bike events, climbing, and adventure racing, I learned the importance of taking care of my feet. Cowman was right. Many times I have forgotten this advice and have paid the price. Feet will take us to new challenges and adventures, but only if we make the conscious choice to care for them

As I eased into the sport of adventure racing in 1998, the proper care and preparation of my feet became even more important as the days of nonstop pounding took their toll. As an ultrarunner, I cared for my feet. As an adventure racer, I experienced a sense of helplessness because I could control only my feet—yet I had three other teammates to worry about. If even one teammate drops out due to bad feet, or any other reason, the whole team is disqualified. Our feet get us from the start to the finish, so we need to give them the best possible care.

Problems with one's feet are commonplace in all adventure races. Adventure racers, ultrarunners, runners, walkers, hikers, thru-hikers, soccer players, and other athletes all need to know how to care for their feet—it can be the key to success. Some of us do extreme events, others more casual pursuits; some do long multiday events, while others head out for only a few hours. No matter how rigorous the outing, proper conditioning of our feet, picking the best footwear, learning what our feet need to stay healthy during an event, and knowing how to fix problems are all part of being successful in any sporting activity and maintaining your success for years to come.

This third edition of *Fixing Your Feet* explains in an easy-to-understand, straightforward way what has taken me 23 years to learn. I learned the painful way. You can learn the easy way—by reading this book, which answers all the questions I once had.

Dan Barger
Primal Quest Expedition Adventure Race Director & Founder
Ultrarunning Grand Slam Record Holder 1998–2002
Adventure racer and ultrarunner

Dedication

This third edition of *Fixing Your Feet* is dedicated to all athletes who have taken the challenge to have fun in their chosen sport. As they train, play, and race, they stress their feet, often to the extreme. When they struggle with their mind telling them to go and their feet telling them to stop, they will find the ideas and tips in this book become important. This book is for them.

Acknowledgments

Special thanks go to the athletes who have shared their experiences and contributed their ideas on foot care. They make this book come alive.

I would like to thank Denise Jones, the Badwater Blister Queen, for her interest in fine-tuning taping methods used by runners and her willingness to be a good listener for my ideas about foot care.

I thank my wife, Kathie, for her continued patience through another rewrite and research process, and my son, Scott, who after one of my 12-hour track runs, gave me the original idea for the first edition of this book.

Thanks to editing by Kate Hoffman, book design by Emily Douglas, and the cover design by the staff of Wilderness Press, this third edition takes *Fixing Your Feet* to a new level of professionalism.

Contents

Fixing Your Feet

Introduction

*"One thing is for sure, when one's feet hurt …
it definitely gets one's attention."*
—Denise Jones, the Badwater Blister Queen

Whether we are walkers, runners of short- to marathon-length events, ultramarathoners, adventure racers of one-day to multiday events, casual hikers or thru-hikers of the long trails, soccer or tennis players, it is our feet that propel us toward our goal. They are our primary means of transportation. Too many of us know how the pain of blistered feet, a turned ankle, or other foot trauma can destroy our motivation to continue in an activity no matter how much our minds prod us to continue.

Out of problems come solutions. My motivation to write this book arose from my personal foot problems and seeing and hearing the horror stories of athletes who suffer as a result of their foot problems. I have cut the socks off a runner's feet at mile 92 of a 100-mile run and seen the skin fall off the bottoms of both feet. I have helped runners who completed a 100-mile run and could hardly walk because of the terrible condition of their feet. I have seen the macerated skin on the feet of runners who fail to take care of their feet through an ultramarathon, and I have watched the grimacing faces of adventure racers as their teammates tried to repair their horribly blistered and battered feet. I have watched as well-meaning crews and teammates have tried to repair the feet of their fellow athletes and as well-meaning aid-station volunteers have tried their best to fix the feet of athletes in their events. In all of these examples, the athletes, crews, and teammates have tried their best based on their limited knowledge of what to do, and most often have done well. But often there is a better way or other options—and they can be found in the pages of this third edition of *Fixing Your Feet.*

If there is one thing I have learned about footcare in the 6½ years since I wrote the first edition of *Fixing Your Feet,* it is that there are lots of foot problems and more than one solution for each problem. When I meet athletes with interesting stories, I am motivated to keep writing about feet. Here are three of their stories.

The first story belongs to Dude:

> I never get blisters. I don't get them in boots, and I don't get them in running shoes. I don't have to toughen up my feet, even if I have been sedentary for months. In my humble opinion, some people's feet are tough as nails and they never get blisters, and other people's feet are literally "tenderfoots" and they get blisters no matter how much they try to toughen them.
>
> I have a friend who runs ultras with me all the time. I usually run one really long run every two weeks and run about 3 miles every other day between the long runs. Conversely, he takes long runs twice per week and typically runs farther than I do, and also runs more like 6 to 9 miles per day between his long runs. When we do ultras, he gets blisters and I don't. Therefore, I believe that some people are lucky and some are not.

The second story comes from Lisa Smith:

> I used to get really bad feet. Since I started using Hydropel and CoolMax socks, I have not gotten any blisters. In one summer I have

done 157 miles through Death Valley in 125-plus heat, plus three 100s: Western States, Old Dominion, and Leadville. I also think having your mechanics looked at by a top foot doctor and having custom insoles made if your biomechanics are off helps as well.

The third is from David Hannaford, a sports podiatrist and ultramarathoner. In the foreword to the second edition of this book, he wrote the following:

> As I was limping over the last sand dune on the last day of the seven-day Marathon des Sables in the Moroccan Sahara desert, I thought of John's advice about foot protection. I was losing a toenail which could have been avoided had I heeded his advice about larger shoes in extreme heat. I thought I knew better. After all I have two silver buckles from the Western States 100-Mile Endurance Run, and being an experienced sports podiatrist, I already fit my shoes roomy. But, as I looked around me, my little injury paled in comparison to the hundreds of runners limping to the finish with feet much more damaged than mine. Most of these foot problems could have been avoided with proper care.

As these three stories illustrate, the common saying is true: We are each an experiment of one. Dude never has problems, Lisa has found a solution to past problems, and David is always looking for new learning experiences. In my humble opinion, taking care of your feet becomes a matter of educating yourself about the best components to put around them. In *Fixing Your Feet,* there are many solutions to every problem.

So, there is hope. With the advanced products offered today, athletes need not suffer from problem feet. With the proper education and choices about foot care, most of the limping athletes could come back next year and play well—without problems—or at worst with problems that pale in comparison to their former ones.

There are no shortcuts to finding what works. What works for one runner's feet may not work for another runner. The foot-care efforts of one hiker or adventure racer may work wonders for him or her but cause you problems. This book offers information that has been well tested by experienced athletes: runners, triathletes, adventure runners, hikers, and backpackers. If you study the information and apply it to your specific foot problems, you will determine what works for you by trial and error. There are hundreds of tips in this book, but the bottom line is that you need to find which ones work for you. Try one. If it doesn't help, try another. Remember, though, that what works for you today may not work for you tomorrow. But by doing your homework, you'll be closer to solving your foot problems.

Two words sum up the advice in this book: *proactive* and *reactive*. Preventing foot problems is being *proactive*—working to solve problems before they develop. When problems develop, everything becomes *reactive*—working to solve an existing problem. Being *proactive* takes time up front. Being *reactive* takes time and resources often when they are not available or when using them may jeopardize the outcome of the event.

No matter what your sport, this book can help your with your feet. Whether you are a walker or 10K runner, marathoner or ultrarunner, overnight hiker or long-distance thru-hiker, tennis or soccer player, triathlete or veteran multisport adventure racer, this book can help you understand how to keep your feet healthy.

Foot Fetish

My feet are runner's feet;
a little rough around the edges,
with black nails on the toes where I have nails at all
Lovingly decorated with bright colors.

My toes are warriors, of a sort.
They carry the entire continent of my body on adventures
and rise to challenges that could crush them.
Some days they are worn and calloused,
but they are strong and fierce adversaries for the
rocks they overtake.

My arches are the springboard of my soul.
They give me lift with every step I take
and cushion all my landings.
They are always ready
when I want to jump for joy.

My heels respond when the shepherd
of my spirit nips at them to run.
They strike again and again,
to thwart frustration,
to redeem the day.

My feet are runner's feet;
a little rough around the edges,
but they are strong
and they are willing
and oh, I love them.

—Lisa Butler, Ultrarunner

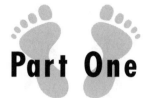

Part One

Foot Basics

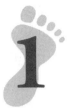

Seeking Medical Treatment

The information and advice given in this book is provided to athletes to use in their efforts to resolve foot problems. Not all foot problems or injuries will be resolved successfully by following the tips or using the products mentioned in this book.

Never ignore an injury. Pushing through an injury or returning to your sport too soon after being injured can lead to additional injuries. You do not want to turn a temporary injury into a permanent disability. Too often athletes rely on self-diagnosis rather than consulting with a medical specialist. If during or after running or hiking you have persistent foot problems or recurring pain that you cannot resolve, you are advised to seek medical treatment from a medical specialist who can provide his or her medical expertise for your problem.

Sometimes these specialists help at events. Dr. Dennis Grandy, the former podiatry director of the Western States 100-Mile Endurance Run, has treated the foot problems of hundreds of runners. He says he has seen "many conditions that were treated 'on the spot' with no medical reference ever being available. Blisters, although very common, are usually overlooked and often cause the runner to drop from the race."

Dr. David Hannaford is a sports podiatrist to many Olympians, ultrarunners, and other endurance athletes. Dr. Bill Trolan has served as medical consultant to adventure racing teams, fixing many participants' feet. Each of these doctors has treated many, many athletes whose success in runs, hikes, and adventure races can be jeopardized due to foot problems. Consider yourself fortunate if you can learn firsthand from a medical specialist.

Primary Medical Specialists for Feet

ORTHOPEDISTS are orthopedic surgeons, experts of the joints, muscles, and bones. This includes upper and lower extremities and the spine. Look for an orthopedist that specializes in the foot and ankle. The American Academy of Orthopaedic Surgeons and the American Orthopaedic Foot and Ankle Society can provide referrals.

PODIATRISTS are doctors of podiatric medicine (DPM) that work on the feet up to and including the ankles. They specialize in medical and surgical problems including foot diseases, deformities, and injuries. The American Podiatric Medical Association and the American Academy of Podiatric Sports Medicine can provide referrals.

If you have chronic foot problems, or you are uncertain what your feet are trying to tell you through their pain, consider consulting a podiatrist or orthopedic surgeon. Listen to your whole body and especially your feet. Be attentive to when the pain begins and what makes it hurt more or less. Then be prepared to tell the specialist about the problem, its history, what you have done to correct it, and whether it worked or got worse.

There is a wide range of skill overlap between orthopedists and podiatrists. Each can treat most of the same foot problems. When searching for a medical specialist for your feet, talk to doctors about their training, experience, and whether they have a specialty field. Each of the two specialist fields has doctors who specialize in sports medicine. Weigh this information when making a decision about who to turn to for help. Additionally, a variety of other specialists can provide assistance in strengthening, alignment, rehabilitation, and footwear design and fit.

Foot Specialists

PEDORTHISTS work with the design, manufacture, fit, and modification of shoes, boots, and other footwear. Pedorthists are board certified (C-Ped) to provide prescription footwear and related devices. They will evaluate, fit, and modify all types of footwear. The American Orthotics and Prosthetics Association and the Pedorthic Footwear Association can provide information and referrals.

SPORTS MEDICINE DOCTORS specialize in sports-related injuries. They are typically doctors of internal medicine with additional training in sports medicine. When treating athletes with lower-extremity injuries that do not improve with their initial treatment, they may refer the athlete to a podiatrist or orthopedist. Most are members of the American College of Sports Medicine (which does not provide referral services).

PHYSICAL THERAPISTS are licensed to help with restoring function after illness and injury. Most work closely with medical specialists. Physical therapists use a variety of rehabilitation methods to restore function and relieve pain: massage, cold and heat therapy, ultrasound and electrical stimulation, and stretching and strengthening exercises. The American Physical Therapy Association can provide referrals.

ATHLETIC TRAINERS are licensed to work specifically on sports-related injuries. Rehabilitation methods may be similar to physical therapy but can additionally focus on maintaining cardiovascular fitness while injuries heal. The National Athletic Trainers' Association can provide referrals.

MASSAGE THERAPISTS work with athletes in reducing pain and tightness in muscles, tendons, and ligaments—the body's soft tissues. The American Massage Therapy Association can provide referrals.

CHIROPRACTORS are doctors of chiropractic medicine who specialize in the alignment of the body's musculoskeletal system. Muscle imbalances, and pelvis, back, and neck pain are often treated by a chiropractor. Some may specialize in sports injuries. Two organizations, the American Chiropractors Association and the International Chiropractic Association can provide referrals.

When the time comes to seek medical attention, ask others in your sport for referrals or look in the Yellow Pages. If you have a choice, choose a sports medicine specialist over a general doctor. For contact information for the professional organizations mentioned above, check "Medical and Footwear Specialists" on page 323.

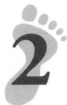

Sports & Your Feet

Running, hiking, and adventure racing place extreme demands on our feet. Soccer, football, and court sports stress the feet and ankles with their quick changes in direction and sudden stops. Skiing and snowshoes encase our feet in unforgiving hard boots that also stress our ankles. The surfaces we play and compete on vary from dirt, rock, grass, asphalt, and concrete to wooden courts, tracks, snow, and ice. Every sport offers wide ranges of difficulty. We challenge ourselves with ultramarathons on trails or roads. We test our limits in adventure races under extreme conditions. We tackle the multisport fun of duathlons and triathlons. Whatever our sport, our feet take a beating.

A run may be a relatively short road 10K or a grueling ultrarunning event of 100 miles with over 40,000 feet of mountainous ascents and descents. It may be in a short- or medium-length duathlon or triathlon, or a longer Ironman or Ultraman Triathlon. There are also further extremes: 24-, 48-, and 72-hour runs, six-day runs, and 1000-mile races. The terrain may be paved roads, tracks, fire roads, trails, cross-country, or any combination. You may run without any gear, with a single water bottle, or with a fanny pack or lightweight backpack loaded with extra socks, food, and water bottles.

A hike may be a day trip with a daypack, an overnighter with a midweight 40-pound backpack, or a ten-day high-Sierra trip with a pack that tips the scales at 65 pounds. You may be a traditional backpacker with a full-size pack that carries all the comforts of home, a fastpacker with a

30-pound pack, or an ultralight backpacker with a 16-pound pack. Typical backpackers may cover 6 to 10 miles in a day, fastpackers may cover 20 miles, and ultralight backpackers can easily cover 30 miles or more. The hike duration may be a night in your local hills, a week in the desert, three weeks in the Sierra, or several months on the Appalachian Trail or the Pacific Crest Trail.

Adventure racing includes events with names like Primal Quest, Eco-Challenge, the Raid Gauloises, or the Beast of the East. These are typically competitive team races with up to five participants who must all finish together. Combining sports disciplines like trail or cross-country running, mountain biking, rappelling, climbing, kayaking, canoeing, horseback riding, swimming, glacier climbing, and others, these races pose challenges along an often unknown course with constantly changing terrain. Many are multiday events over distances up to 450 miles. In these team events, the whole team is only as fast as the feet of its slowest member. Robert Nagel, one of the world's best adventure racers, recalls his experiences in the 1996 Extreme Games: "Our team had a strong and growing lead when my feet caused us to grind to a crawl. We continued, barely, losing over 12 hours in the process, but still managed to take third place." He remembers that ESPN was continuing to show tapes of his feet 16 months after the event! After that experience, he worked hard to perfect a foot-care regimen that would prevent such a disaster from happening again.

Most sports require considerable use of the feet, and participation in these sports requires an athlete to keep his or her feet happy and healthy. Many of these athletes have learned the finer points of keeping their feet in shape. They rely on the many sources of conventional wisdom about foot care, but while much of this wisdom is good, the best advice often comes from athletes who through trial and error have found unique solutions for the prevention and treatment of their foot problems. I think Ronald Moak, an Appalachian Trail thru-hiker (1977) and Pacific Crest Trail thru-hiker (2000), sums it up best: "I would like to think that after 30 years of backpacking, I'd have solved the little dilemma of my feet. But, alas, I'm not that naive." Ronald has the right idea—it's good to listen to all forms of advice and then try different things. Don't be afraid to go against conventional wisdom. Just because it didn't work for others doesn't mean it won't work for you.

Sport Similarities

What do the sports discussed above have in common? Foot-stressing sports have many similarities. They pound the feet, stress the joints, and strain the muscles, often to unnatural extremes. They may take place over a day, yet often are done over several days, or even a week or more. While athletes participate in these sports, their feet become highly susceptible to hot spots, blisters, and problems with toenails, stubbed toes, bruises, sprains, strains, heel spurs, plantar fasciitis, and Achilles tendinitis. All of these sports can be more enjoyable by solving these common foot problems.

Runners put considerable weight on their feet with each step. Though hikers move slower than runners, they often find their feet stressed by the weight of a fully loaded fanny pack, lumbar pack, or backpack. Adventure racers may stress the feet faster in shorter events or longer over multiday events in which they compete in multiple sports and carry the special equipment they require. The longer multiday adventure races often tax the feet more than we can imagine with the regular exposure to water, constantly changing adverse conditions, and lack of time to do proper foot care.

In Roland Mueser's book *Long-Distance Hiking: Lessons from the Appalachian Trail*, he describes what he found when he surveyed hikers:

> Problems with feet were endemic. Half of the hikers experienced blisters at the start; many of these were attributed to thrusting tender feet into stiff, heavy boots. During his first few days in Georgia, one hiker was forced into a hospital for an entire week with so many serious blisters that his trip was terminated. And even later when hikers' feet became toughened, the combination of rain, heavy boots, and wet socks meant trouble for one out of five on the trail. One foot-troubled backpacker reported having seven blisters at one time. And more than one hiker, squirming out of boots, was horrified to see socks soaked with blood.[1]

Studies have shown that "carrying heavy external loads, (i.e., a heavy backpack) during locomotion appears to increase the likelihood of foot blisters."[2] In addition, the type of physical activity performed is a factor in the probability of blister development. As we intensify our activity and as the duration of the activity increases, frictional forces are increased. Heavy loads, high-intensity activities, and long-duration activities are what we do as runners, hikers, and adventure racers. In our events, most of us experience at least two of these three stressors. Ultrarunner Suzie Lister typically experiences few problems with her feet while running ultras. However, when she participated in the 1995 Eco-Challenge, the added weight of a pack on her back and the multiday stresses of adventure racing caused many problems with her feet: blisters-on-top-of-blisters and swollen feet.

The similar stresses among sports make the preventive maintenance and treatments for blisters and other foot problems necessary for all sports. This book approaches the different disciplines—running, duathlons and triathlons, hiking and backpacking, and adventure racing—as one and the same when dealing with one's feet. Proper foot care is the most important variable for a successful outing.

Differences in Terrain

The terrain is an important part of your running, hiking, and playing environment. While a flat, smooth, and resilient surface is ideal, most of us do not have that luxury. Nor do many of us want that type of surface. Most runners spend the majority of their running miles on roads, while most hikers spend their time on trails. Variations from our normal running or hiking surface can produce problems as we compensate for uphills, downhills, concave surfaces, or irregularities of the surface. Be aware of compensations in your stride or gait due to changes in the surface.

Dirt & Trails

Dirt and trails provide a soft running and hiking surface. Trails or fire roads can open new vistas to the adventuresome athlete. Some trails are well groomed, while others are barely maintained. Soft dirt trails provide excellent shock absorption and can be a good surface to use if recovering from an injury.

Whether running or hiking, pay close attention to trail hazards like rocks, roots, wet leaves, mud, and other potential hazards, any of which can cause a turned ankle or a fall. On rainy days, slippery mud and grasses can present problems with footing. Watch for uneven terrain, roots, and holes on grassy sections of trail. Trail dust, dirt, pebbles, and rocks can be kicked up into the sock or between the sock and the shoe. These irritants can cause hot spots, blisters, or cuts. Gaiters worn over the shoe or boot tops can help prevent this problem (see "Gaiters," page 129).

Doing trails while wearing a backpack presents the added problem of maintaining one's balance with a top-heavy load while negotiating rocks, roots, and uneven trail. Attention to your footing can help prevent a turned ankle. Striding uphill stretches the Achilles tendons and the calf muscles, and makes the pelvis tilt forward. Going downhill increases the shock impact to the heels when landing and tilts the body backward. Constantly going up- and downhill may also cause problems with toes, toenails, heel pain, plantar fasciitis, and more.

Grass

Grass is a forgiving surface and a great choice if you are prone to road-impact injuries. Be careful of uneven grassy areas, holes from burrowing animals, the slipperiness of wet grass, and the occasional rock.

Roads

Road running is the mainstay of most runners. The asphalt surface of most roads provides a softer surface than concrete sidewalks. However, roads have slanted, concave surfaces curving down towards the sides. The concave surface puts more stress on the downward side of your shoes and your body. The foot of the higher leg rotates inward, while the foot of the lower leg rotates outward. Spend a few minutes on your favorite roads to check the angle of their curve and be aware of it. Avoid prolonged running on slanted surfaces or at least spend equal time on both road shoulders. Keep your eyes open for potholes and manhole covers. Of course, the biggest hazard to roadrunners is vehicles. Where possible, run opposite the flow of traffic and safely to one side of the road, and choose roads with wide shoulders.

Concrete & Sidewalks

Concrete is approximately 10 times harder than asphalt. While the surface is usually smooth, your bones, muscles, and connective tissue get hammered. This surface can cause foot, leg, or back pain through the jarring of the joints. Care must be taken to watch your footing on sidewalks to avoid the tapered edges of driveways and drop-offs at curbs. The use of good, cushioned shoes and gel insoles can make concrete bearable. Doing high mileage on concrete can lead to overuse injuries.

Courts

Court play is usually on either asphalt or wood. Tennis courts may be indoors or outdoors. Basketball, racquetball, and other indoor sports are usually on wood. While an asphalt or wood court surface is hard and unforgiving, the main foot stresses for athletes playing on them issue are sudden, quick movements and sudden starts and stops. Cushioned or motion-control shoes, depending on your feet, will protect your ankles. A good shoe fit, coupled with moisture-wicking socks and insoles, will prevent hot spots and blisters.

Sand

Walking or running on sand is hard work. Though sand is soft, its surface is not typically flat. Your heels may sink in more than the forefoot and the uneven sand may cause a turned ankle. If you have access to a beach, try to stay near the water on the wet and fairly hard sand.

Snow & Ice

Walking or running in the snow or on ice can be challenging. There may be snow on top of a layer of ice. Your shoes cannot make good traction unless they have been modified with small screws or special traction gear. Falling is a hazard and muscle pulls can be common as you slip or slide.

Tracks

Most of us at some time run on tracks. True, they can be boring. Running in circles, actually in ovals, lap after lap after lap after lap may not be your idea of a good run, but there may be a time for it in your running schedule. A track allows us to calculate with accuracy how fast we are running. I have used a track for occasional speed workouts. Prior to my first 24-hour track run, I spent three hours running at a local high-school track to "get a feel" for the repetitiveness of track running.

The continuous running in one direction stresses the outer leg, so change direction every now and then. Dirt tracks should always be checked for ruts and uneven surfaces that could cause you to trip. Running in the outer lanes is less stressful when rounding the curves.

Conditioning

Conditioning means more than getting your body in condition. It also means getting your feet into the best shape possible for your sport. Your feet will respond to training in the same way your legs respond. Increasing your running or hiking time by increments will allow your feet time to adapt to the added stresses of the additional mileage. Doubling your mileage too quickly will likely lead to potential problems. If you are working up to a marathon, an ultra, or a multiday hike, do back-to-back training days to work your feet into their best possible condition.

personal experience

"In 1991, I walked through immigration in the old Stapleton International Airport in Denver, wide-eyed and fresh from Australia and sporting some nice neat size 9 wingtips, comfortably encasing my soft corporate toes. Ten years later I am outgrowing my somewhat less than nimble size 11 trail shoes, with nary a hope of ever squeezing back into my old wingtips. This rather dramatic change in foot size is due entirely to conditioning. In 1984, when I started adventure racing in Australia, I had a size 8 shoe, but the intervening 18 years spent running and hiking around for prolonged periods with a pack on my back has resulted in a physiologic adaptation.

"This is really just conditioning. The same effect can be seen in farmer's hands, which grow to quite unusual sizes over decades of manipulating heavy machinery and tools. It is not uncommon to walk into a bar in the Midwest and see the little old farmer, neatly shrunk inside his once tight-fitting Wrangler jeans with absolutely enormous gnarled hands nursing a beer.

"So, to get these nice big, abuse-proof peds, spend some time on them. Lots of time. So much time that they hurt real bad. I don't usually say this, but in the case of feet, no pain, no gain. Don't go out and get bloody blisters, but do go out for those really long hikes, with a pack stuffed with baguettes, Camembert, bottles of red wine, and the kitchen sink and really abuse your lower leg structures. Work the crossword every day and you will get good at it, wield a hammer all day and you will get calluses on your hands, hike with a heavy pack for hours and you'll get bigger, tougher feet!"

—Ian Adamson, adventure racer

Brick Robbins was an adequately trained runner when he started his thru-hike of the Pacific Crest Trail, but he quickly found running had not conditioned his feet. The extra weight of a backpack caused additional stress to his feet. After 100 miles his feet were sore and bruised. By the time he reached Idyllwild—another 70 miles down the trail—he had "killer" blisters that took another 270 miles to heal. Although his feet were in good shape from running, they needed additional conditioning for the weight of a pack. There are no shortcuts to conditioning your feet. Your feet will become conditioned to longer distances by gradually increasing your mileage.

When Karen Borski thru-hiked the Appalachian Trail in 1998, she had very few foot problems. A year before the thru-hike, however, her feet were so out of shape that after an 8-mile day hike they would be riddled with huge blisters on the sides of the heels. Wearing a pack, she found that after only a few miles blisters would begin to develop on the soles of her feet, usually the balls of the feet where the main pressure is felt. Karen recalls she was "so frightened and worried about these blisters that I was afraid I would not be able to thru-hike." To fix the problem, she first bought new boots that were slightly too large so that during the course of a hike, as her feet naturally swelled, they wouldn't become too tight and rub. Then she started hiking with a pack every weekend. After hobbling around for most of the following week nursing these awful blisters, she would go out and do it again. When calluses finally began to develop, she took up running on the weeknights, both to get her body in shape and to help toughen her feet. Karen found that developing large calluses on her feet before starting the AT hike helped so she did not have many problems with feet along the trail.

So, what is the best way to condition your feet? Your feet must be conditioned to endure the rigors and stresses of your chosen sport or sports. Train in race conditions in the shoes and socks you will wear on race day. Do short hikes with a pack on your back before taking off to tackle a multiday hike. Use a wobble board to strengthen your ankles. Toughen your feet with barefoot walking. Work up to distances that you will tackle in your event. Work out the kinks; find the best shoes and socks for what you will be doing. Learn how to trim your toenails and reduce calluses. Discover the proper insoles that provide support to relieve your plantar fasciitis or heel pain. Strengthen your toes and ankles. In short, do your homework before you head out to tackle the big one. Your feet will thank you.

Biomechanics

Many athletes who have participated in extreme sports have learned firsthand how one minor problem can be magnified over time and eventually have major consequences. Typically this happens when a blister affects the gait, a backpack's weight throws off balance and stance, or stressed or weakened muscles cause an imbalance in the body's mechanics. Every athlete has different strengths and weaknesses, different degrees of flexibility, and different muscle skills and body types. These factors affect the way we walk, run, and move. Add on a fanny pack or backpack, or put a flashlight in one hand and a water bottle in the other hand, and our biomechanics change. Each time your foot lands, it absorbs about 2.5 times your body weight. For every mile you travel, your feet hit the ground around 800 times each.

The Importance of Alignment

You all know the foot bone is connected to the ankle bone, and the ankle bone is connected to the leg bone. True, correct alignment of all those bones at the joints keeps you moving relatively pain free now, and prevents many degenerative changes down the road. Total body alignment is essential to the success of any athletic activity.

Even more important to the healthy functioning of the feet and their ability to carry you through life is the spine—the very specific focus of chiropractors. The spinal cord carries sensory and motor information from your feet (and everywhere else for that matter) to your brain and back again. If one of the vertebral bones is even slightly misaligned or fixated, it can affect the communication lines and your feet and brain can be broadcasting misinformation. The joints of your feet and particularly your ankles contain nerves called proprioceptors that send messages about the changes in terrain you are walking, standing, or running on. The brain then interprets and makes the miniscule changes in every joint in your body, from the tilt of your skull to the tuck of your tailbone, to keep you upright.

Chiropractors come in many styles. I recommend one who specializes in sports chiropractic and who adjusts extremities as well as the spine. Those chiropractors are certified in orthopedics and can design a rehab program of strengthening and stretching. Always get referrals from other runners and make sure the chiropractor is a good fit for you.

—Pam Adams, chiropractor

Maryna, a holistic practitioner who was part of the medical team at the Canadian Eco-Challenge, emphasizes how your whole leg and, indeed, your whole body needs to function in a unified, integrated way. She saw a lot of blisters caused by legs being out of alignment in various places from hips to knees to ankles. Misalignment causes radical changes in all phases of your footfall from strike to breakover to push off. Problems can work from the legs down or from the feet up. An understanding of biomechanics will help us visualize the cause and effect.

Understanding Biomechanics

Biomechanics is the study of the mechanics of a living body, especially the forces exerted by muscles and gravity on the skeletal structure. The foot, which includes everything below the ankle, is a complicated but amazing engineering marvel. With an intricate biomechanical composition of 26 bones each, together they account for almost one-quarter the total number of bones in the entire body. Thirty-three joints make each foot flexible. About 20 muscles manage control of the foot's movements. Tendons stretch like rubber bands between the bones and muscles so that when a muscle contracts, the tendon pulls the bone. Each foot contains more than 100 ligaments that connect bone to bone and cartilage to bone and hold the whole structure together. Nerve endings make the feet sensitive. With each step you walk or run, your feet are subjected to a force of two to three times your body weight, which makes the feet prone to injury.

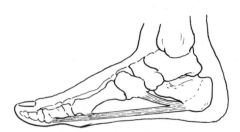

Side view of the bones of the foot.

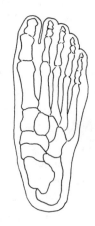

Top view of the bones of the foot.

The big toe, commonly called the great toe, helps to maintain balance while the little toes function like a springboard. The three inner metatarsal bones provide rigid support while the two outer metatarsal bones, one on each side of the foot, move to adapt to uneven surfaces.

Your feet are each supported by three arches. The transverse arch runs from side-to-side just back from the ball of the foot. This is the major weight-bearing arch of the foot. The medial longitudinal arch runs the length of the instep, flattening while standing or running, giving spring to the gait, and shortening when you sit or lie down. The lateral longitudinal arch runs on the outside of the foot. Both longitudinal arches function in absorbing shock loads and balancing the body. These three arches of the foot are referred to singularly as the foot's arch.

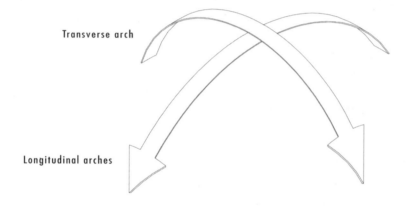

Transverse arch

Longitudinal arches

With a basic understanding of the foot's construction, it becomes increasingly important to be aware of how we affect our body's biomechanics. At some point in training for an event, we need to try to mimic the event itself. Wear the same shoes and socks that you plan on wearing during the event. Wear the same clothes. Carry the same weight in a fanny pack or backpack. Even get out in the same weather. Although we may not realize it, these factors can change our stride, work different muscles, and put pressure on different body parts—including the feet.

Avoiding Biomechanical Problems

The body lines up over the foot. When the foot goes out of alignment, the ankle, knee, pelvis, and back may all follow. Analyzing the way we stand, walk, and run helps a podiatrist or orthopedist determine whether we have a mechanical misalignment and how it can be corrected. He or she will also want to see your running shoes to analyze the wear patterns on the soles.

An example of biomechanics is the functioning of the foot's arch. A low arch, or flat foot, typically occurs when the foot is excessively pronated, turning it inward. A high arch supinates the foot, rolling it outward. Both of these structural variations can cause knee, hip, and back pain. When one arch flattens more than the other arch, that inner ankle moves closer to the ground. That hip then rotates downward and backward causing a shortening of that leg during walking and running. The pelvis and back both tilt lower on the shortened leg side and the back bends sideways. The opposite leg, which is now longer, is moved outward towards the side that puts added stress on its ankle, knee, and hip. The shoulder on that side then drops towards the dropped hip. All of these are compensations as the body adapts. Muscles, tendons, ligaments, and joints are stretched to their limit. The body is out of alignment.

The stresses on our bodies can result in inflammation, often the cause of foot pain. Running on unbalanced and uneven feet may result in fatigue. Fatigue gives way to spasms that may cause a shift in the shape of our feet. Corns, calluses, bunions, spurs, and neuromas may develop when joints are out of alignment.

Do not fall into the trap of drawing erroneous conclusions about your injuries or the type of shoes or equipment that you need for your running style. A podiatrist or orthopedist should check pain associated with running. Heel pain that we try to resolve with a heel pad may not be caused by a heel problem but by arch problems. This in turn may throw off the biomechanics of the body's alignment. If you begin a run and right away experience knee pain, you most likely have a problem with the knee. If the pain comes after running for a while, it is most likely not a knee problem but a biomechanical problem. Likewise, you may think because you are a heavy runner you need a shoe with lots of cushioning. Based on that decision, you buy a cushioned shoe, the most cushioning insoles, and wear thickly cushioned socks. But, in reality, what you may need is a stability control shoe. This is where the help and expertise of medical specialists comes in. They are trained to determine biomechanical problems.

In 1991, Craig Smith and his brother set out to hike 300 miles of the Continental Divide Trail. With training and planning done, they started with heavy packs that tipped the scale at almost 58 pounds each. Two days and 22 miles later, Craig had developed severe pain in both knees. Forced to abort the trip, they cached as much gear as possible before starting back. With Craig's knees wrapped with torn T-shirt strips, it took them four days to backtrack the 22 miles. It took several weeks of conditioning therapy before he could finally walk without a limp. Craig now packs lighter, does exercises that focus on strengthening the knees, and uses a walking stick on downhills. He could have easily been a victim of biomechanical problems that centered in his knees.

Remember that most athletes have foot problems or become injured by doing too much, too soon, and too fast. To avoid biomechanical problems, use proper footwear, pace yourself, do strength training, and train in the gear you will use in your event.

Form & Health

As long as you have good form, whether running, hiking, paddling, or biking, you stand a better than average chance of not injuring yourself due to a

biomechanical problem. But let the pack ride wrong on your back so you lean to the side, weak abs make you lean forward, tired arms cause your shoulders to drop, or spent quads cramp up, and your body is tossed out of alignment. This will ultimately work its way down to your feet. As they compensate for your biomechanical problems, your gait and stride change, and your feet develop their own problems.

Your best bet is to maintain good form by thinking smart and training wisely, whatever the discipline. Make sure your shoes are not worn down—replace them before they lose their support and cushion. Wear good insoles to balance the foot and provide good heel

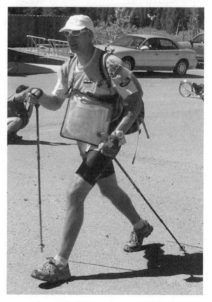

Use hiking poles for support and to help the knees.

and arch support and alignment. Strengthen the ankles and knees with specific exercises. Do upper body exercises to strength your abs, back, and shoulders for carrying your pack. Work your arms so they can help maintain balance and proper form. Learn how to tape a sprained ankle or turned knee. Condition yourself in incremental stages without huge jumps in mileage or extremes. Train with the gear you will use in an actual race—building up to appropriate weights rather than carrying everything all at once. Use hiking poles for support and to help the knees. Learn your body's weak links and find exercises to strengthen those muscles and joints.

Every one of us, at one time or another, can fall victim to biomechanical problems as we race to extremes. Train smart and race smart, and you can stay healthy, starting with your feet.

CONDITIONING PRODUCTS

POLES can be used to hike farther and more comfortably, absorb shock, keep your knees healthy, and help maintain balance. Walkers, hikers, backpackers, and adventure racers have discovered the benefits of poles. Made of either aluminum or carbon fiber, many models offer antishock support and carbon tips. Poles are made by Black Diamond, Komperdell, Leki, MSR, and REI. Typically called hiking or trekking poles, they can be found in sporting goods and camping stores.

REEBOK'S CORE BOARD helps build strong core muscles of the stomach and lower back, which will help your stride and develop flexibility and balance. The Core Board flexes on a rubber center post that lets it twist, tilt, and rotate; this forces your body to recruit core muscles to balance or hold a position. The board's flexibility can be changed as you adapt to the conditioning. Reebok also offers a set of three how-to videos of core conditioning programs. **Reebok, (800) 733-2651, www.reebok.com**

WOBBLE & ROCKER BOARDS can be used to improve balance and strength, retrain injured muscles, improve muscle memory, and build core strength. Fitter First has the most comprehensive line of boards, and training charts and programs. **Fitter International, (800) 348-8371, www.fitter1.com**

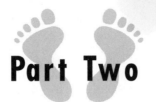

Part Two

Footwear Basics

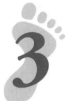

The Magic of Fit

Fit is key. Again, repeat after me: "*Fit is key.*" It is not everything, but without properly fitting shoes or boots, your feet will encounter many problems that can initiate many others. If your footwear is too loose, your feet will slide around, creating friction. If your footwear is too tight in certain areas, your feet will experience excessive pressure. Wearing too loose or tight footwear will change the biomechanics of your foot strike, which in turn will affect your gait and throw off your whole stride and balance. This will stress your tendons and ligaments. When your feet and toes are pinched in too-tight shoes with socks that make the fit even tighter, the blood circulation is reduced. To top it all off, you will endure aches and /or pain, and will be more tired from dealing with all of the above. Sounds like fun, right? Unfortunately many athletes have resigned themselves to this type of process. They go out strong for as long as their feet last—which in many cases is not as long as they had hoped and often is well before the finish line or the end of their journey. Does it have to happen this way? You decide.

Fit starts with properly fitting shoes with a quality insole. No matter how good your socks are or how well you apply tape or how good any other component is, if the shoes fit incorrectly, you will have problems.

In *Advanced Backpacking*, Karen Berger makes a good comment on the fit of boots—and the same advice applies to any sport shoe. "Like most marriages, the mesh between boot and foot is not always a good match. If you look at the feet of several people, you'll undoubtedly see a range of bumps and bunions, arches and anklebones—all of which are encased in the same hard leather cage. It takes a bit of time, accommodation, and softening for boots and feet to settle into a comfortable routine."[3] Because our feet are so different, many factors go into achieving in a good fit.

Rich Schick, a physician's assistant and ultrarunner, believes the key to getting the proper size shoe is the insert: "If the foot does not fit the insert, then the shoe will have to stretch to accommodate the difference or there may be excessive room in the shoe, which can lead to blisters and other foot problems." He thinks there is too much confusion about straight lasts, curved lasts, semicurved lasts, and so on:

> You don't need to know any of this if you use the insert to fit your shoes. The same holds true for the proper width of shoe. Simply remove the insert from the shoe and place your heel in the depression made for the heel [in the insert]. There should be an inch to an inch and a half from the tip of your longest toe to the tip of the insert. None of your toes or any part of the foot should lap over the sides of the insert. If they do, is it because the insert is too narrow or is it because of a curved foot and straight insert or vice versa? The foot should not be more than about a quarter inch from the edges of the insert either. This includes the area around the heel, or the shoe may be too loose. Check to see if the arch of the insert fits in the arch of your foot. Finally, if all the above criteria are met, then try on the shoe. The only remaining pitfalls are tight toe boxes and seams or uppers that rub.

Many shoe and boot companies suggest specific models that are best for certain types of activities and sports, and for certain types of feet. They do this because many shoes are made for a specific type of foot—and many people have feet that will work better with one type of shoe than another. Look for the buyer's guides in the magazines of your sport. Runners can find shoe reviews in *Runner's World, Trail Runner, Running Times,* and *UltraRunning.* Backpackers and hikers can check out *Backpacker* magazine's boot reviews, and *Outside* magazine's Buyer's Guide for helpful information.[4] Adventure racers and triathletes can benefit from these reviews as well as the occasional review in *Adventure Sports, Triathlete,* and *Inside Triathlon.* For information on shoe reviews and gear review sources, see page 321 in the appendix.

Other sport-specific magazines may offer similar reviews. Many Websites are now posting reviews, and some even offer reader comments/reviews.

Can there be more than one shoe that is right for your feet? Are there perfect shoes? Christopher Willett went through four pairs of shoes on his 2003 Pacific Crest Trail thru-hike (2600+ miles) and bought them as he went. Wearing size 15 in running shoes, he didn't really have the option of buying from an outfitter along the trail. He would call or use the Internet from various towns along the way and have new shoes and socks sent up trail. He started in Brooks Adrenaline GTS and liked them in the hot 563-mile Southern California section. He wished the next shoe, the Asics Eagle Trail, had a more protective sole but liked the tread. While the New Balance 806s were structurally good, he felt they had a poor tread design and they are the only shoe that he would not wear again. He finished the last 670 miles in the Asics Gel Trabuco V and liked their durability and tread. Would one of the shoes have worked for his whole thru-hike? If they had been the NB 806s, the answer would be no. Probably any of the other three would have worked the whole way, but Chris might have had problems sticking with one shoe given the varying weather and terrain of the trail. Even the most perfect shoe can have small issues: breathability, tread design, cushioning, sole protection, and so on. Each of these issues can make them perfect for one set of conditions and wrong for another.

Buying Footwear

Intelligent EVA, AHAR, Impact Quotient Technology, Grid, SpEVA, Fusion Technology, Arch Lock, XT1200 Super Abrasion, DuoMax Medial Post, Cross Deck, IGS, I-Beam, Over-the-Top, HRC, CRM, DuoTruss System, Instep Support Device, Trusstic System, TRB Shank; the list is almost endless. It's not enough that we had a Grid. We also have a 3D-Grid, a T-Grid, a Visible Grid, a Non-Visible Grid, and a Dynamic V-Grid. What are these? Are we talking about automotive technology, computer terms, building codes? No, they're all acronyms and terms that shoe companies are using in their effort to convince you and me what we need in our next pair of shoes. (Most of these acronyms or terms are registered trademarks of their respective shoe companies.) The above list is from only three shoe companies.

Think of how long and confusing the list would be if it included all the shoe and boot manufacturers.

Buying shoes has evolved to a level of complexity never before seen. Buyers have to study the latest issue of their favorite running, ultrarunning, adventure racing, triathlete, or outdoors magazine, or try to read through the materials posted on manufacturers' Websites to comprehend the language they're speaking. Does Impact Quotient Technology really matter to you or me? Does IGS really guide my foot "from heel to toe in a much more natural, comfortable stride"? I know what a truss is, so is a Trusstic System something similar?

We're not buying a car, just a pair of shoes. But the complexity of the selection process recently was turned up several notches. If you want to find the best shoes, you now have to read the fine print—and understand what the fine print means. Many of the acronyms and terms above are puzzling unless you read further. Some of the shoe company's Websites are very helpful, offering images and understandable explanations of what these things mean. But some are downright useless.

The bottom line: We need to find a shoe that fits well, lasts more than a few miles, and doesn't rub us the wrong way. And after we buy the shoes and find that we love them, we hope they don't discontinue them in six months when the new models are released. There is something to be said for brand loyalty. I have it and I suspect many of you also do—especially when you've found a pair that fits well.

Personally, I would never buy shoes from any source without trying them on, and walking in them, running a short bit, or using them on an incline board. I prefer to frequent my local running stores, walking stores, and hiking/outdoor stores. I avoid, like the plague, the chain stores that often have shoes that I have never heard of—even if they are from major well-known companies. I get mail order catalogues from companies that sell all types of shoes and related gear, and I often check out Internet sites where shoes are also sold. If I know a particular shoe and know that it fits my foot, I might buy from one of these, but with rare exceptions, I buy from my local store. I value the service, the help with fit, the evaluation of my old shoes, and their look at my gait as I try out the new shoe. My bottom line: I want a shoe that works on my foot, a shoe that fits as well as possible, and a shoe that's right for whatever sport I throw at it.

Buy your shoes wherever you want, but remember, fit is one of the most important elements of using your shoes and boots without problems. Your local shoe store is dedicated to providing you with high-quality choices in shoes and service you can't get through mail order. There is more than one pair of shoes for your feet. There may be a half dozen models that will fit well. The experts at your local store will help you select several brands and models to come up with a good final choice.

Know Your Feet

With knowledge of biomechanics and your specific foot type, you can make a better choice than shopping blindly. When shopping for shoes or boots, try on several different pairs from several different companies. This will help you identify those that initially feel good versus those that just don't feel quite right. Knowing how different shoes and boots fit your feet will help in the final selection.

A biomechanically efficient athlete lands on the back outside of the heel and rolls inward (pronation) to absorb shock. The foot flattens as the motion moves forward, rolls through the ball of the foot, and rotates outward (supination) to the push off. Over-pronation is the inward roll of the foot as you roll off the heel.

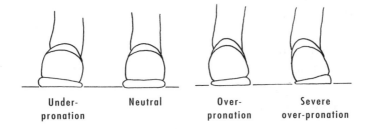

Under-pronation   Neutral   Over-pronation   Severe over-pronation

There are two main schools of advice for preparing to purchase shoes. One school suggests asking a friend to watch or even to videotape your feet as you walk or run to determine how they land and your general form. This information and the wear patterns on your old shoes can help you decide whether you should look for shoes that compensate for under-pronation, over-pronation, or severe over-pronation, or whether you can get by with shoes for neutral pronators. Use this information to select shoes from one of four categories: flexibility trainers for under-pronators, stability trainers for over-pronators, motion-control trainers for severe over-pronators, and neutral trainers for neutral pronators.[5]

Another school suggests that you first consider your running and bio-mechanical needs, including your most common running surface, and then select one of five categories that best matches your needs: motion-control, stability, cushioned, lightweight training, or trails. Secondly, determine whether your foot type is normal, flat, or high-arched (discussed below). Use this information to select shoes from within that category.[6]

Take your old shoes with you when you shop for new shoes. The wear patterns on the soles can help you or the salesperson determine how you run and the best shoes for your running style. Normal wear is on the outer heel and the across the ball of the foot. Pronators show wear both on the outer heel and the inner forward side of the shoe. Supinators typically show wear on the heel to the forefoot along the outer edge of the shoe.

The key to a good fit in running shoes is to know your foot type. To determine this, walk on a hard surface with wet, bare feet to see your imprint.

The Three Arch Types

FLAT-ARCHED FEET leave an imprint that is almost completely without an inward curve at the arch. Looking down their leg, these athletes will typically see their feet turned outward like a duck's feet. They will typically do best in a semicurved or straight last shoe that offers good stability and/or motion control. They are often over-pronators. The use of an arch support is usually helpful.

NORMAL-ARCHED FEET leave an imprint that shows the forefoot and heel connected, but with an inward curve at the arch. Standing and looking down their leg, these athletes will see their ankles and feet follow the vertical line down their lower leg. These athletes will typically do best in a semicurved last shoe since they are generally efficient in their gait. They might benefit from a cushioned or stability shoe with moderate control features.

HIGH-ARCHED FEET leave an imprint that shows the forefoot and heel connected by a very narrow curve at the arch. If your feet are turned inward, you will typically do best in a curved last shoe with good cushioning. Athletes with high arches are typically under-pronators and should avoid motion-control shoes.

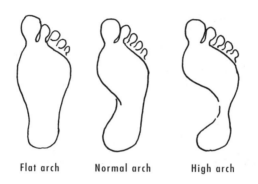

Flat arch   Normal arch   High arch

Shop around until you find running shoes that feel right on your feet. A correct fit will help in blister prevention. Valerie Doyle remembers her fight to beat blisters. When she learned how to buy shoes that fit properly, she found they solved her blister problem. The same applies to fitting boots. Studies have found that tight footwear can increase the forces exerted by the shoe or boot on the foot, increasing blister probability, while loose-fitting footwear increases the movement of the foot inside the shoe or boot, causing increased friction forces on the foot, which in turn increases blister probability.[7]

Walk in the shoes or boots for a while to be sure they are comfortable and do not have any pressure points. Some shoes and boots will be higher at the ankle and may put pressure on your foot. Others will not bend at the same forefoot and toe point, making an uncomfortable heel to toe transition or pinching the toes. There may also be a seam inside the shoe or boot that rubs your foot and creates pressure and a potential blister. Pay close attention to the overall fit.

You may find shoes that fit well with one exception. The toes may pinch or you may have corns or bunions that create pressure in specific areas. Some runners will cut slits into the side or the toe boxes of shoes to provide a better fit. Other runners will actually cut out a portion of the shoe over the problem area. If you do this, be careful not to sacrifice the integrity of the shoe. Be aware of an additional problem this may cause: Dirt and small rocks can easily get into the shoe and lead to hot spots and blisters.

If you have narrow or wide feet, consider shopping for shoes or boots that offer variable lacing capabilities. These shoes and boots will have lace eyelets that are not lined up in an up-and-down row but spaced horizontally farther apart. See "Lacing Options" (page 136) for information on how to lace for different types of feet.

The American Academy of Orthopaedic Surgeons gives suggestions for buying shoes. Foremost, they remind us that shoes should always conform to the shape of your feet; your feet should never be forced to conform to the shape of a pair of shoes. Their suggestions apply equally well to buying boots.

Components of a Good Fit

Fit can be achieved with simply a little common sense and a bit of luck. Out of all the shoes and boot to choose from, there is more than one brand and style that will fit your feet well. When you find them, buy several pairs. Rotate them, but save the best pair for the race or event you are training for.

Apply common sense when trying on the shoes or boots.

Common Sense Tips for Trying on Shoes

- ☐ Try on and fully lace both shoes.
- ☐ The shoes should feel comfortable. You should feel no discomfort in any part of the shoe's fit.
- ☐ Feel around the inside of the shoe for rough spots where the parts of the uppers are stitched together.
- ☐ Your feet should have some room to breathe and swell.
- ☐ Your toes should have plenty of room to move and wiggle, and the toe box should not be too short in height or length. Aim for at least 1/2 inch to 1 inch of space between your longest toe and the front interior of the shoe.

☐ The tops of your feet should not be pinched when the shoes are laced properly.

☐ Be sure the shoe's counter (the part that wraps around your ankle and heel) does not rub your foot wrong. Your heels should be snug in the heel counter of the shoe and should have little up and down movement. There should be a firm grip of the shoe to your heel, but not too firm.

☐ The arch of each foot should be supported, but the shoe arch should not be too high, or too far backward or forward, for your foot type.

☐ The shoes' shape (last) should be comfortable and not overly curved or straight for your foot type.

☐ The shoes should fit well with the same type of socks you will be wearing in your training and/or race event.

☐ The shoes should flex well for the type of terrain you will encounter and at the right point of your foot. This will help provide support to your ankles and prevent uncomfortable heel to toe transition or pinching of the toes.

☐ The shoes should provide adequate protection for the bottom of your feet from rocks and uneven terrain.

☐ The fit of the shoe should come from the shoes themselves, not from tying the laces.

☐ The laces should stay tied the way you like them without coming undone.

☐ The shoes should have outsoles for the type of event or race you will be doing. They should help keep your feet in place inside the shoes.

☐ If the insoles that come in the shoe are weak and flimsy, replace them when you are buying the shoes—get a pair that provides support and cushioning.

☐ If you will be using orthotics or special insoles, make sure they fit in the shoes without pushing your feet too high in the shoes' uppers or too far forward.

Tips for a Good Fit

Whether buying shoes for running, hiking, court sports, soccer, or golf, it is important to get a good fit. When you purchase footwear, consider the whole picture, not just the shoe or boot you hold in your hand. Your footwear must work with your choice of socks, insoles, and orthotics (if your wear them), and also with the activity you will be using them for. Hiking boots that feel okay when you walk around the store may feel different when you get home and try them when carrying a 30- to 40-pound pack on your back.

Here are some suggestions for getting the best possible fit:

- Use shoe buying guides as just that—do not eliminate a shoe from your consideration until you have tried it on.

- Try shoes in a range of prices—don't save a buck at the expense of your feet. The differences between several pairs of shoes can be amazing.

- Judge a shoe by how it fits on your foot, not by the marked size.

- When going to try on or buy shoes, take a pair of your socks along rather than rely on the store's basket of socks that have been on who knows how many feet.

- Do not buy a pair assuming they will fit better later unless they are leather boots. In most cases, today's shoes and boots require no breaking-in period.

- Have your feet sized each time you buy new footwear. Measure both sitting and standing to determine your elongation factor.

- Fit new shoes to your larger foot.

- Try on shoes at the end of the day, preferably after running or walking, because your feet normally swell and become larger after you have been standing and sitting all day.

- Today's running shoes and lightweight hiking shoes are very well made and in most cases will wear as well or better than many of the heavier boots.

Footwear purchasers frequently forget to allow enough toe space when buying shoes and boots. When your foot is in the shoe, the arch naturally flattens. Since your heel is held in place by the shoe's counter, your foot can only move forward. If the shoe does not have this bit of extra space in the toe box, the toes become cramped. Toenail problems, blisters, and calluses may develop.

Customizing Your Footwear

When you shop for shoes or boots, run your fingers around the inside to determine whether there are any rough spots, overlapping or raised seams, or other potential pressure points that could cause hot spots or blisters. These may be able to be rubbed flat or softened. Ask the store for another pair to determine if the spots are common to that style or just one particular shoe or boot. If these spots are common to that particular shoe or boot, your choice is to have the shoe modified by a show repair shop or find another style that fits correctly.

The contour around your heel and ankle has to be smooth from the base of your foot all the way up to your ankle or the top of your heel. If a shoe or boot has any ledges, ridges, or extrusions around the ankle or heel, they will rub into your feet and potentially cause a problem. These extrusions may be there due to stitches, extra foam, or by design. Hiker Buck Jones has had two such bad experiences with heel and ankle rubbing. In the first, he was an hour into a short hike in his new pair of trail running shoes when he discovered that the ledge in one had made a hole in his sock and was working on his ankle. He recalls, "I applied duct tape and moleskin to my foot and also patched the shoe with duct tape and moleskin so that the ledge was minimal." He was able to finish his hike with little more wear on his foot. His second experience was with a friend who was a beginner hiker. Shortly after starting the hike, she was bothered by a hot spot. The boot had a stitch around the heel and it was causing a blister. He applied duct tape and moleskin on the foot and under the void of the stitch. By mending both the foot and the shoe they were able further further skin damage. Now before Buck buys a pair of shoes, he checks for a bad design around the heel and ankle area.

If you have difficulty finding quality shoes that fit your particular type of foot, consider searching for a certified pedorthist. They are trained to work on the fit or modification of shoes and orthotics to alleviate foot problems caused by disease, overuse, or injury. He or she may be able to modify your footwear, internally or externally, for a better fit. Look in the telephone book or ask your orthopedist or podiatrist for references. Information on the Pedorthic Footwear Association can be found under Medical and Footwear Specialists in the appendix (see page 323).

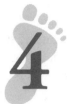

Footwear & Insoles

Many people consider footwear as simple basic equipment that takes little thought. Yet the war against foot problems can be lost over ill-fitting shoes, boots, or socks that cause blisters or insoles that are not right for your activity. Choose your footwear based on which sport you will be doing, the terrain expected, and your level of experience. Find the right shoes or boots and the right socks based on what feels right and fits correctly—not by price. Tom McGinnis, who thru-hiked the Appalachian Trail in 1979, makes a good observation: "Good boots and bad socks can be miserable. Cheap boots and good socks can be a dreamland." This chapter focuses on types of running shoes, sport shoes, hiking boots, and insoles. Sandals are briefly discussed because they are becoming popular. Socks play such a large role in preventing problems that they are discussed at length in their own chapter.

Our feet are unique. Yours may look similar to mine, yet they are as different as our fingerprints. Although our feet may fit into the same size and shape of shoe or boot, our feet actually mold into the footwear differently. Corns, bunions, susceptibility to blisters, toe length, the type of arches, and the shape of our feet are just a few of the factors that affect the fit of our footwear. Even how we react to and recover from the stresses of running and hiking is important in choosing shoes and boots.

Only you can determine what type of footwear you need to wear. Certainly runners wear running shoes, but there are many types of running shoes. Hikers and adventure racers have many choices in hiking boots, but many make the choice to wear running shoes instead of boots. Many of the top teams racing the Eco-Challenge wear running shoes for the whole event, even on snow and ice and while wearing crampons. Just remember the "ifs." If you are used to hiking in running shoes, if your ankles are strong, and if the shoes provide the necessary support while wearing a pack, then running shoes may be right for you.

When shopping for shoes or boots, try on several different pairs from several different companies. This will help you identify those that initially feel good versus those that just don't feel quite right. Knowing how different shoes and boots fit your feet will help in the final selection. When going to buy new shoes, you may have a preferred shoe, sometimes based on magazine ads or on the recommendations of others, but buy only those that fit best. Whichever type of shoe you wear, be sure to train in them. Never wear a new pair in a race. Always break them in before the race.

Socks vary in thickness, and changing socks can change the way your feet fit inside your shoes. When trying on shoes, wear the same socks when trying on shoes that you wear during races. When buying new socks, be sure they will not alter the fit of your shoes. If your new socks make your shoes fit tighter, you may be able to fix this with new slightly thinner insoles.

TIP: Best Friend to Worst Enemy

Whatever sports shoes you wear, remember to inspect them regularly for problems. Frank Sutman was on the second day of a six-day 80-mile backpack trip when one boot's outersole split from the midsole to the ball of the foot. He suffered through four days of flapping sole, picking up pebbles, rocks, sticks, and even being tripped up. The moral of his story: Check your boots and shoes before major activities and periodically to keep small problems from becoming major inconveniences. Split outersoles, ripped or torn fabric that lets dirt and rocks into the shoe, cracked heel counters that create folds in the inner heel material, or broken laces retied into a bothersome knot over the top of the foot are all preventable.

The Anatomy of Footwear

By understanding the parts of a shoe or boot, you can make informed choices about which running shoe, cross-trainer, or boot is best for your sport—and for your feet. The parts of a shoe are fairly common, regardless of what kind of footwear you are looking for.

Parts of a Shoe

- The shoe's **COUNTER** is the part that wraps around the heel of the foot.
- The **HEEL** is the back bottom of the shoe.
- The **INSOLE** is the inner insert on which your foot rests. These are typically interchangeable.
- The **OUTERSOLE** is the shoe's bottom layer.
- The shoe's **SHANK** is the part of the sole between the heel and the ball of the foot.
- The **TOEBOX** is the tip of the shoe that shapes and protects the toes.
- The **UPPER** is the top of the shoe that surrounds the foot.

Running Shoes

There are many sources of information about which shoes may be the best for you. The five main sources are the shoe companies, local running stores, magazines and catalogues, running friends, and the Internet. Recognize the difference in the quality of help available at some chain shoe stores in shopping malls versus stores that specialize in running shoes and equipment. A specialized footwear store usually has personnel who are athletes themselves and can watch you run, look at your old shoes, and recommend specific brands of shoes and styles based on what they see and your answers to their questions.

To understand running shoes, you need to be aware of their construction. The first construction component is the *last,* the form over which a shoe or boot is constructed.

Running Shoe Last Patterns

BOARD last shoes have the shoe's upper material glued to the shoe's board, which runs the length of the shoe. This generally produces a fairly rigid and stable shoe.

COMBINATION last shoes have the shoe's upper material stitched to either the forefoot (slip-lasted) or the rear foot (board-lasted). This design offers additional stability at either the foot plant or the toe's push-off.

SEMICURVED lasts are molded straight towards the rear foot while having some curve towards the forefoot. This mold provides stability and flexibility.

SEMISTRAIGHT lasts are built to curve slightly from the toe to the heel. This provides some flexibility and a high degree of stability.

STRAIGHT last shoes are built along the shoe's straight arch to provide maximum stability.

SLIP last shoes are made with the upper material stitched directly to the midsole without a board. This offers maximum flexibility.

Basic Categories of Shoe Construction

NEUTRAL shoes are made for the runner who has good biomechanics and would be categorized as a neutral pronator. These shoes generally have a good blend of flexibility and stability.

FLEXIBILITY shoes are made for runners who are under-pronators, who have foot motion towards the outside and need a shoe that offers more shock-absorbing pronation than their body can deliver.

STABILITY shoes offer high stability and cushioning. Midweight or normal-arched runners without motion problems who are looking for good cushioning typically use these shoes. These runners usually over-pronate slightly beyond neutral and need a shoe with extra medial support. Most are built on a semicurved last.

MOTION-CONTROL shoes provide the most control, rigidity, and stability. Heavy runners, severe over-pronators, flat-footed runners, and orthotic users often choose these shoes. They are typically quite durable shoes, but they are often heavier. Most are built on a straight last and offer the greatest level of medial support.

TRAIL RUNNING shoes usually offer increased toe protection, outsole traction, stability, and durability. Runners who run mainly on trails usually use these shoes.

CUSHIONED shoes are those with the best cushioning. These are typically used by those who do not need extra medial support and by high-arched runners. Most are built on a curved or semicurved last.

LIGHTWEIGHT shoes are typically made for fast training or racing. These come with varying degrees of stability and cushioning and can be worn by runners with few or no foot problems. Most are built on a curved or semicurved last.

Buying Running Shoes

Running shoes are changing rapidly. The major shoe companies roll out new designs twice a year. Shoes now offer midsole air, gel, and tube chambers, springs, recoil plates, Gore-Tex and other membrane fabrics, breathable liners and mesh outer fabrics, and better support and stability. More models have been released for trails as this market as grown many times over.

Once you buy a new pair of shoes, wear them around the house to be sure they fit well and are comfortable. If you sense problems, return the shoes for another style or type. Even the same shoe model that you have worn in the past can have minor design changes in a new release. Wear them for a while until you are sure they fit well.

Shoe designs are always changing. Often our favorite shoes disappear from the shelves and we find ourselves forced to make new choices. Do your homework, study the shoe reviews and the ads, talk to your running friends, and try on various styles. Good stores will let you run in them. Ultrarunner Orin Dahl once found that his favorite shoes were no longer offered. Instead of the old shoes, Nike offered a new type of "air" shoe. He bought the shoes and began running in them. The new shoes were not as flexible in the forefoot causing his heel to pull up and out of the shoe. To his dismay, he developed blisters at the back of his heels. He recalls how he turned the shoes over to the Salvation Army and began a search for a different pair. He has no doubt that the shoes were good shoes, but they were just not right for his feet and running style. As you look for shoes, remember that not every pair of shoes is right for your feet.

"I *personal experience*

did ten 100-mile runs in 1999: Rocky Raccoon, Umstead, Massanutten, Old Dominion, Western States, Vermont, Leadville, Wasatch, Angeles Crest, and Arkansas.

"I really didn't have too much of a problem with my feet that year. The Rocky Raccoon (the first race) is where I had the most trouble. It was 80 degrees and very humid, and I wore my last year's shoes, which were size 11 (my normal size). Since the shoes were a bit worn and [my feet had] some swelling due to the humidity, I had several blisters between my toes. After the run, I drained them with a pin and then pretty much forgot about them.

"I then bought some Asics 2040s and Montrail Vitesse shoes in size 12. I always wear double-layer, blister-free socks. The rest of the [year], I had very few blister problems. The only consistent blister problem was with the Montrails. If I didn't put duct tape on the balls of my feet, they would develop blisters. They also rubbed on the outside of my left big toe. I did not need any tape with the 2040s. Even at the hot and humid Vermont 100, I had little problem with blisters, [and what I problems I did have were] mostly as a result of wearing the Montrails. On rare occasions, I would get a small blister on the inside of the big toe on my right foot.

"I never put anything on my feet. I do, however, use Succeed electrolyte caps. This has helped me with stomach distress (I only drink water or, late in the race, Pepsi). I am sure that [the caps] also help with the blistering. I think experience has a lot to do with blisters. The more races I run the tougher my feet become."

— *Jeff Washburn*

Sports Shoes

By sports shoes I mean any shoes specific to your particular sport. These may be soccer, football, baseball, or climbing shoes, or even cross-trainers.

Even military boots can be considered in this category—the requirements for getting a good fit are the same.

When shopping for these shoes, apply the same basic principles that you would for other athletic shoes. Try several different brands and styles. Try them on wearing the socks you will wear during the activity. Lace them up and be sure they hold your heel, that your toes have wiggle room, and that they feel comfortable.

Many sport-specific shoes such as those for soccer have a simple thin insole with virtually no arch or heel support. These can lead to arch problems, metatarsal pain, blisters, and more. The first thing I would do when I find a shoe that fits well is to replace the standard flimsy insoles with a good supporting insole—but do this when buying the shoes to make sure they are big enough to accommodate the insoles.

Climbing shoes are meant to fit close to the skin. These are often worn without socks, so be sure there are no irritating seams that can cause blisters. If you will wear thin socks with the shoes, take them along when shopping for shoes. One problem area in climbing shoes is the tight toe box. If you have Morton's toe, hammer toes, bunions or corns, or other toe problems, be aware of how the tight fit will affect that condition. Understanding any preexisting foot problem will help you make an informed choice of shoes. Each of these conditions is discussed later in this book.

Military boots may not offer much in the way of selection, but you need to be aware of many of the fit issues discussed in the next section about hiking boots. Irritating seams, poor heel fit, thin insoles, toe boxes that are too narrow and too short, and boots that are not correct for the shape of your feet can lead to long-term problems. If given a choice in boots, try on several to get the best fit possible. Again, as with most other shoes, replace the insoles. Then choose a good moisture-wicking sock.

"O *personal experience*

n my feet, I wore a liner sock, SmartWool socks, and Wellco jungle boots with an enhanced cushioned midsole and Vibram-type sole. I coated my feet with BodyGlide. This combination had worked very well for me in training, with no blisters, and so I anticipated no problems. During the competition, however, I developed hotspots fairly early on the bottom of my feet. By mile 5, I was pretty sure that some of the hotspots had turned into full-on blisters; my suspicion quickly proved right. At about the 5¾-mile mark, I picked up a trot as the course came off a dike. As I did so, I felt an excruciating pain on the bottom of both heels. I realized two things: my feet were going to hurt a lot, and quitting just wasn't an option . . . Somehow I did manage to qualify for the new unit.

"As an experienced triathlete, I made some right choices. However, with the combination of a heavier 45-pound pack, gravel roads, liner socks that were too tight, and unseasonable warm and humid weather, my feet were doomed from the start.

"I don't know that anybody teaches foot care to subjects in basic training. A lot of information is passed along through informal instruction in the ranger and infantry communities, but it may not be up to date and may not reflect lessons learned from people like endurance athletes and adventure racers. The sad thing, however, is that if you showed up to a non-infantry (or non-special ops) unit on the morning that they'd decided to do a road march, you'd see some frightening equipment choices and personal preparation. There's very little foot-care knowledge in many combat support units. It makes me shudder just to think about it."

— *army ranger, describing a 12-mile forced march that was part of the selection process for an elite special operations unit*

Hiking Boots

My first pair of hiking boots was all leather, with thick Virbram soles. They laced all the way to my calf and seemed to weigh as much as my loaded backpack. Times have changed and so have hiking boots. They fit better and are easier on your feet. Running-shoe technology has had a positive influence on hiking boots. Insoles, molding, padding, and midsole and outersole advances have made many of them as comfortable as lighter-weight boots. A recent ad by bootmaker Sorel claimed, "Any boot can repel water. Ours will actually suck the sweat off your pinky toes." As technology advances, many bootmakers, like Sorel, will offer moisture-control systems to wick perspiration away from your feet. Gore-Tex fabrics are commonly built into boots for moisture transfer. Lacing systems are also changing for the better.

Kent Ryhorchuk has the right attitude about hiking footwear:

> When it comes to budget, I would not be stingy on anything related to your feet. Your feet will hurt badly enough without having to deal with blisters and chafing. Bad feet stopped or hobbled many people the year I hiked, mostly due to blisters—even some experienced Appalachian Trail hikers. The shoe-and-socks system I use for footwear is Montrail Vitesse shoes, flat Spenco green insoles, Birkenstock blue footbeds over the Spenco insoles (to control my metatarsal problems), Smartwool low-cut hiker socks, and Fox River X-Static liner socks. It took several years of hiking, trail running, and adventure racing to figure this out, but I went from getting blisters all the time to hardly ever getting blisters at all. The point is that I spent a lot of time on it, not that this system is necessarily right for anybody else. Everybody's feet are different.

Many hikers have been converted to using the newer lightweight boots. These are usually as flexible as running shoes and carry many of the running-shoe benefits of fit and comfort. Because of their flexibility and construction, many of these boots require very little or no break-in time. I completed an 8½-day, 221-mile ultralight backpack of the John Muir Trail in regular running shoes. Unless you are used to hiking or running trails in running shoes while wearing a backpack, I do not recommend them for backpacking. Since I did the John Muir Trail in 1987, boots have changed. Today, I would consider a trail-running shoe or lightweight boot for the same hike.

Check out some of the features of new hiking boots at your local store. Many boots offer a combination of features: lighter weight, breathable uppers, high-traction and long-lasting outersoles, improved lacing systems, flexible footbeds, stable and cushioning midsoles, wider toe boxes, and Gore-Tex fabric incorporated into the uppers. Some boot companies, like Merrell and Vasque, have developed what they call their "hiking boot last," which is designed to be snug around the heel and arch, and with a roomy toe box. Both offer three different insoles for a better fit, and the use of different thicknesses of socks and the number of pairs worn can adjust the fit even more.

Boots falls into three basic categories: lightweight hiking (for trail hiking and light loads), midweight hiking (for on/off trail hiking and light backpacking), and heavyweight hiking (for on/off trail, heavy loads, and multiday trips).

Before you go shopping for boots, determine the type of hiking you will be doing and how much support and protection you will need for the weight you will carry. Then, look at the various features of different boots in each of the three categories. Finally, shop accordingly, but do not rule out a certain type of boot until you try them on your feet. A boot that pinches or rubs in the store will not feel better when you are out on the trail. Rob Langsdorf suggests taking time to really test a new boot before leaving the store:

> I usually wear mine around the store for an hour or more before deciding to take it. It takes time but consumes less time than having to return it or having to spend lots of time treating blisters. Then, break new boots in by wearing them around the house, to work, church, etc., before going out on the trail. Begin with easy hikes before starting off on a long trip. Only when they feel good on a short hike are they ready for a longer one.
>
> I had a friend who bought a pair of boots, but didn't break them in because she felt that wearing them around the house wasn't the feminine thing to do. She ended up with major blisters after 6 to 7 miles. Buy the end of our 15-mile weekend backpack she was ready to throw the new boots away and swear off ever backpacking again— all because she didn't want to look funny wearing her boots in town.

Some boots will soften and become more flexible with forceful flexion of the soles and uppers, hand-working a waterproofing solution into the leather, or mechanical flexion of the uppers at a shoe shop. If your boots are too stiff, try one of these three methods.

Ed Acheson made several painful discoveries when he hiked the Pacific Crest Trail. Before he began his trip, he switched to a new pair on a sales-person's recommendation. The boots were too much boot for him and a half size too small—the salesperson told him they were sized larger than most. Ed remembers for the first 20 days having "more blisters than the number of days I had been out." To compensate for the blisters, he changed his gait, which in turn gave him knee problems. Before he could get new boots, he was forced to cross the Mojave in tennis shoes. He suffered for years from problems he attributes to the wrong boots.

And even after you have broken in your boots, be sure they still fit after not wearing them for a while. Wear them for at least one getting-reac-quainted walk before going on a major hike. Your feet may have changed, and they may need to get readjust to the boots before a long hike.

Buying Hiking Boots

Before buying new boots, understand how they are changing. Boot designs are offering waterproof, breathable Gore-Tex liners, thinner leather for better hot-weather hiking, better lug soles for increased traction, lugs that extend up the rounded sides, better insoles, softer uppers for shorter break-in times, snug ankle collars to keep debris out, and more. Boots are being made better, but never buy a pair for their features alone. Buy them because they fit.

Before buying boots, check *Backpacker* and *Outside* magazines (and their Websites) for their coverage on hiking boots. These articles evaluate most brands based on fixed standards while identifying their features and costs. Then check out your local backpacking supply store for the brands and styles they carry. Spend as much time as is necessary to get a good fit. Tell the salesperson what type of hiking you will be doing, for how long, and how much weight you plan on carrying. Try on several pairs of boots by dif-ferent companies. Use your own socks. Walk in the boots. Squat in them. Look for a pair that fits right from the start and grips your heels. Take out the insoles and look at the boot's construction. Find the pair that fits and feels better than the others. Purchase a high-quality boot made for hiking rather than lighter weight boots sold for general-purpose street wear. These fashion-statement boots will not hold up under the stresses of heavy trail use. Utilize the experience of the personnel of your local camping and back-packing stores to help you make a wise decision, but realize the final deci-sion is yours based on how they feel on your feet.

Remember that the boots you select will each be picked up and put down many times each day. Hiking 12 miles each day would equate to about 25,000 steps[8], day after day. Feel the weight of your boot and think about each step. Heavier boots are not always the best. True, they may provide more ankle stabilization, but you could get more benefit from a lightweight boot and proper ankle and foot-strength conditioning before the hike. Ray Jardine, who has hiked the Pacific Crest Trail three times and the Appalachian and Continental Divide trails each once, estimates that each 3½ ounces off a pair of boots could add about a mile to a day's hiking progress.[9] A review of one store's boot selection showed weights for a pair of boots ranging from 1 pound 9 ounces all the way to 3 pounds 9 ounces. Selecting boots that weigh 10½ ounces less than another pair could mean an additional three miles hiked per day. An educated choice based on boot features, your personal needs, and the terrain ahead is necessary.

If you are planning a several-week hike or a several-month thru-hike on a multistate trail, you will need to buy boots that are larger than normal to accommodate your feet as they become stronger and enlarge to their normal hiking size. Try on boots that are anywhere from one to two sizes larger than normal, which will allow your feet to fit into them properly. If you need to purchase new boots midway through a long trek, be aware of potential problems of breaking in new boots.

Mara Factor has experienced her feet changing:

> Be wary of buying multiple pairs before you start. Most people's feet change significantly as they hike. The shoes you wear day to day will adjust somewhat and continue to fit your feet. New shoes, the same size as the ones you've been wearing for a while, often do not fit. Longer and/or wider sizes are often required after spending a few hundred miles on the trail. I used to be a woman's size 12 before I started long-distance hiking. Now I'm a men's 13 (I can't find women's 14s or 15s). I may be an extreme example, but most people do have some change along the way. It may be worthwhile to plan a side trip or two off the trail to go to an experienced outfitter who can remeasure your feet and make sure the next pair will fit properly.

When you do have problems with your feet, and you usually will at some point, you need to look at the boots and evaluate whether you need to replace them with another boot type and/or style. On long hikes, your feet do enlarge and change. Boots wear out. Over a couple of years your feet may also change. Be open to new styles and features in newer type boots and find the pair that best fits you.

If you are always having problems with your boots and a different set of boots does not help, consider trying a pair of running shoes, preferably trail running shoes. Be aware, however, of the differences. Running shoes do not provide the same degree of ankle support and overall foot protection. While some may prefer the increased ankle mobility of a low running shoe, this choice requires proper strength in the feet, ankles, and legs. My choice to wear running shoes when fastpacking the 221 miles of the John Muir Trail was based on a trial overnight hike with a full backpack and years of running trails. I knew my feet and ankles could handle the stresses of the trail in running shoes, and I did not need heavier boots.

One week into hiking the John Muir Trail, Andrew Ferguson developed a "hellatious" deep blister on the back of his right foot, about 1 ½ inches in diameter. By nursing the blister with Spenco 2nd Skin and tape, he hiked for three days in running shoes before reaching civilization and purchasing a new pair of boots. The red heel bothered him for two weeks and took six months to return to normal. Andrew is now a believer in running shoes for hiking. Many people prefer running shoes instead of boots for hiking.

Sandals

Sandals are a nice alternative to shoes and boots. They are becoming more popular as designs improve to provide better traction, foot control, and comfort. Changing from running shoes or hiking boots into an open pair of sandals can be refreshing. When your feet are tired, hot, or sore, sandals can feel like a small piece of heaven on earth.

Spencer Nelson, who prefers Bite sandals, recommends sandals for some uses:

> I have put in some quality training and races in them to have gotten a feel for their use. I always wear them with socks (usually Smartwool) and have worn them for flat 5-mile runs to 20 miles on trails to day two of the Tahoe Triple Marathon, which had 13 miles of downhill. They are good for my feet, and I will probably get another pair for the following positive reasons. They are very comfortable

and better cushioned than they appear. I don't even notice they are a sandal after four or five minutes . . . in other words the straps and open air feel don't affect me. They are quick to dry on trail runs with water crossings. They keep my feet cool. They feel as good after around 200 miles as they did when I got them. Scree gets in and is easily kicked out . . . honestly! I have not had any problems with stubbing my toes or things of that nature.

Those who prefer the freedom of sandals over constricting shoes may find the Wraptor or the newer Bite sandals to their liking. Teva's Wraptor was the first performance running sandal. Using a patent-pending strapping system and a fusion arch, the sandal offered adjustability, comfort, and control. The strapping system flexes to adjust to the runner's arch and assist in motion control. The newer Bite sandals are made for cool, comfortable use, providing the cushioning, stability, and support of a running shoe in a light-weight, airy sandal.

Wearing sandals while running or hiking takes practice. Small pebbles, gravel, leaves, or other debris can easily work their way underfoot. Shaking the foot or a light kick against a rock will usually knock these loose. Be especially careful of sticks on the trail that could inflict a puncture wound to your exposed feet.

If you wear sandals without socks, the skin of your feet will eventually toughen into calluses. Check the calluses regularly for cracks that can split through to uncallused skin and bleed or become infected. If going without socks, a dab of sunscreen on the toes and tops of the foot will protect from bothersome sunburn. Currently the most popular sandals, from Bite and Teva, do not come in half sizes. This may cause some slippage. Wearing socks could help make the fit better. Another reason to consider wearing socks is that long stints without socks in unsupportive sandals can displace the heel's protective fat pad, which can lead to cracks and fissures in the skin. Some athletes have glued Spenco Hiker insoles onto the sandals, while others use Velcro to secure insoles or foot pads onto the sandal's footbed.

Tired of running shoes that fit him poorly, caused blisters and toenail problems, and seemed to collect dirt, Rob Grant bought a pair of sandals. He used his Teva Terradactyls in a Sri Chinmoy 24-Hour Run. At 100K both small toes were swollen. The next day he ground down the ridge on the footbeds that fits under the toes. This corrected the problem. After putting 405 miles on the sandals, he reports no noticeable wear on the soles or the straps. Rob found that rubbing Vaseline on the inside of the straps helped to soften them. He feels that ankle support in sandals is comparable to that of running shoes. In 2000, Rob changed to the newer Wraptor sandal but found they retained debris in the heel area and it took more effort to clear the problem. Even so, he has used the Wraptors in trail ultramarathons.

SANDAL PRODUCTS

BITE SANDALS are designed for running, hiking, watersports, and walking. Their unique design allows the sandals to accommodate activity-specific insoles or be customized by your podiatrist. Bite offers three types of insoles, for walking, water use, and running. The sandals have a heel cup, arch shank, beveled heel, dual forefoot flex grooves, toe guard, and a multifunction Orthosport outsole with variable-sized traction lugs. Specific models are made to fit women's feet. The Xtension model for running uses Bite's patent-pending Enerflow System to provide the support and comfort necessary for running. The system includes a Phylon midsole for support, a shock pad in the heel to absorb impact, a forefoot spring bar in the toe to provide thrust, and a medial insert for lateral support. **Bite Footwear, (800) 248-3465, www.biteshoes.com**

KEEN FOOTWEAR makes sandals with the protection of a shoe and the comfort of a sandal. The sandals have a toe guard, traction outsole, a wide footbed, and a quick-release drawstring closure. **Keen Footwear, www.keenfootwear.com**

TEVA sandals are for walking, running, and water sports. The Wraptor 2 is made for running. It has a raised toe spring to protect from rocks, roots, and debris; a dual density EVA midsole with a molded shank arch plate; a Heel Shoc Pad; a quick dry upper; and a heavily lugged traction rubber bottom sole. This sandal will work well on trails and roads. With a contour molded, waterproof suede footbed, the sandal would be comfortable in bare feet. **Teva Sport Sandals, (800) 376-8382, www.teva.com**

Hikers and backpackers can benefit from sandals. Jerry Goller backpacked in Merrell or Teva sandals for five years. He reports, "I use them in winter (with SealSkinz and fleece socks) and summer. My feet are actually warmer than when I hiked in boots. They are much more comfortable and, of course, lighter. Stream fording is easier. Ankle support is overrated—sandals work just fine for my feet." Jerry's longest backpack wearing sandals is 800 miles!

Chris Migotsky usually runs 5 to 10 miles in Bite sandals—all on trails with a few rocks and roots and one or two stream crossings, but nothing too severe. "My longest run has been 13 miles, he notes. "I haven't had any problems and always wear socks with them. Because I do some barefoot running on grassy trails I figured the running sandals would make sense for me. I hate feeling constrained in shoes."

When shopping for sandals, try several designs. The straps may rub you wrong. A different style may offer straps that fit better. Some strapping systems require readjustment each time you put them on. If you will be wearing socks with them, be sure they have adequate space for your socks. Look at the soles for adequate traction design. Some designs offer a lip around the front edge of the sandal that can provide a degree of protection from rocks and roots. When fording swift streams in sandals, be aware that the current may unexpectedly catch the sandal, so pay extra attention to your footing.

Insoles

Insoles, sometimes called footbeds, are designed to provide extra support and/or cushioning during running and hiking. Some models are molded to cradle the heel, support the arch, and cushion the forefoot, while others have only an arch support or are flat. Replacement insoles are to be used in place of your shoe's standard insole. Many replacement insoles offer better heel support, shock absorption, energy return, and reduction of friction than the insoles that come with the shoes. Some have a better arch support that will help with flat feet problems. The insoles listed below are typically found in running, camping, and sporting goods stores. Ask to see their product catalogs if their shelf stock is low or if you are looking for a particular type. Some stores offer custom-made insoles that may provide a better fit than a general insole.

There are basically two types of insoles available: foam and viscous polymer. Foam insoles are lightweight and inexpensive, and they retain heat. Their disadvantages are not offering as good impact absorption, and they lose their impact absorbing properties with use. In general, foam is more suited for runners because of the concern about weight. The viscous polymers are a great choice for athletes with sensitive feet or injuries that require protection to the foot's padding. Some insoles offer polymer at the heel and/or forefoot, and the rest is made of foam. This reduces the weight liability of all-polymer insoles.

If you have tried changing socks and other techniques to decrease your chance of blisters, try changing insoles. You may find that a particular brand or type of insole may be better at reducing blisters on your feet. This is usually due to the fabric or components of the insole. Replacement insoles may be sized differently. Be sure to check the fit inside your shoes or boots. An insole that is narrow in the forefoot can create problems as the foot overlaps space between the narrow insole and the side of the shoe. Insoles may be different in other areas also. Some may have a higher arch that will put pressure on your foot, creating blisters. Others may have a narrow heel bed and cause friction where your foot rubs against the top edge of the heel cup. Finding and using the right insole can make a big difference in the overall fit and comfort of your footwear. But insoles are not made to last forever. Check them for breakdown and replace them when necessary. This will depend on how you run and hike, and your mileage.

Replacement insoles are not sold as corrective footbeds. If a particular brand or style of insole is uncomfortable or causes pain, try another type. One brand may fit your feet better than another brand. Some are quite rigid, while others are very cushioned. Try several until you find a pair that is comfortable for your activity. If you purchase insoles and they are too tight in certain areas of your feet, inquire with your local shoe repair shop or a pedorthist about thinning them with a belt sander.

Do not confuse these insoles with an orthotic. Always consult with a pedorthist, orthopedist, or podiatrist if you are having frequent foot problems. Repeated foot pain may be a sign of deeper foot problems that a general-use insole cannot correct. In that case, an orthotic may be necessary to correct an imbalance problem. See the chapter on orthotics for more information on what these can correct and the types available.

INSOLE PRODUCTS

The replacement insoles listed below are a sampling of what is available to the general public. New models and designs are constantly being introduced. Check your local running, hiking, and footwear stores, or the manufacturers' Websites to see what is available. Many of the shoe and boot companies like Montrail, Birkenstock, Merrell, and Vasque also make insoles. Many drug stores and pharmacies also stock insoles such as those made by Dr. Scholl's.

AMFIT CUSTOM-FIT INSOLES are an example of what some stores offer to the general public. They are often used as a substitute for orthotics. AmFit uses a scanned image of your feet to make a custom insole. **AmFit, (408) 986-1232, www.amfit.com**

DRYZ INSOLES help the feet stay dryer and cooler while eliminating odor. The wicking sock liner transports the foot's perspiration and moisture into an inner layer of copolymer foam that absorbs and stores the moisture in a gel-like substance. The gelled moisture dissipates continuously throughout the day and completely when your shoes are removed. The odor-killing agent ReSent and additional ingredients fight the growth of fungi and bacteria. Their sport insoles are engineered for enhanced comfort, cushion, and performance. **Dicon Technologies, (877) 342-6685, www.dryz.com**

FOOTFIX INSOLES are made with a deep heel pocket for stability, a gel heel cushion for minimizing heel pain, and a built-in arch for underfoot support. **Footfix Insoles, (866) 366-8349, www.footfix.com**

HAPAD COMF-ORTHOTIC is a full-length or three-quarter–length insole. Many people have had considerable success with these. For more information, see "Orthotic Products" on page 127.

RXSORBO makes an assortment of replacement insoles. Several designs use Sorbothane visco elastic polymer inlays in the heel and forefoot for maximum foot-strike protection. Other designs use Sorbothane foam in the full insole. **RxSorbo, (877) 797-6726, www.rxsorbo.com**

SHOCK DOCTOR FOOTBEDS incorporate multiple shock absorbing, support, and comfort components to create a foot-hugging performance platform. The

INSOLE PRODUCTS

Ultra, X-Sport, and Xterra models are suited for athletes. **Shock Doctor, (800) 233-6956, www.shockdoc.com**

SOF SOLE by Implus is a line of replacement insoles made with the Implus Cellular Cushioning System. This open-cell material provides superior shock absorption while allowing air and moisture to pass through. Additionally, these insoles contain a biocide additive to retard the growth of bacteria and fungus. Choose from Sof Motion Control, Sof Athletes Plus, and others. **Implus Corporation, (800) 446-7578, www.sofsole.com**

SOLE CUSTOM FOOTBEDS use "heat to fit" technology, as an excellent, inexpensive alternative to custom orthotics. Offered in Regular and the Ultra Cushioning versions, the footbeds have Poron cushioning, a deep heel cup for stability, and an aggressive arch for support. When you heat the insoles in your oven, put them into your shoes, and stand on them, they mold to your feet. **Edge Marketing Sales, (866) 235-7653, www.yoursole.com**

SPENCO makes several lines of replacement insoles. Their Polysorb line offers a molded full-length cushioning system good for shock absorption and energy return. These are made for specific sport application. The Greenline designs are made from closed-cell neoprene. A moldable arch support can be heated with hot water and shaped to the foot for support, comfort, and stability. A gel line is planned. **Spenco Medical Corporation, (800) 877-3626, www.spenco.com**

SUPERFEET footbeds are made in two systems: Trim-to-Fit and CustomFit. Their corrective shape and design offer a stabilizer cap that provides excellent support and stability to the bone structure of the foot, allowing the foot muscles to function more efficiently. The Trim-to-Fit insoles come in five color-coded designs for specific activities and footwear. The six CustomFit designs are fitted at stores with staff trained in their fit system. **Superfeet Worldwide, (800) 634-6618, www.superfeet.com**

TEN SECONDS makes a variety of impact absorption insoles for sports shoes and support insoles for those needing more support. **TenSeconds, (800) 438-5777, www.griffinshine.com/tenseconds**

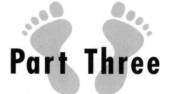

Part Three

Prevention

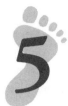

Making Prevention Work

The 6th Law of Running Injuries:

Treat the cause, not the effect.

Because each running injury has a cause, it follows that the injury can never be cured until the causative factors are eliminated.

—Tim Noakes, MD, *The Lore of Running*[10]

im Noakes' sixth law of running injuries must be heeded—any running injury can be cured *only* after the cause is found and eliminated. All of us who run, hike, or adventure race at some point have problems with our feet or sustain foot injuries. The prevention chapters are numerous and lengthy because many factors contribute to foot problems and injuries, and for every factor, there is a preventive measure that can reduce or eliminate it. Prevention is the key to saving your feet. Dave Scott, a good friend and ultrarunner, put the foot problem in proper perspective: "When you don't take care of your feet during a long run or race, each step becomes a reminder of your ignorance."

"Be Prepared." That's the motto of the Boy Scouts. "Be prepared for what?" someone once asked Baden-Powell, the founder of the Boy Scout movement.

"Why, for any old thing," he answered.

It's very easy to relinquish our responsibility for preparedness and let someone else dictate what we should do. We tend to listen to those whom we look up to and to those who are more experienced. In many ways this is okay, and it is often the way it should be. However, only you can determine what works for your feet.

Knowing your prevention options is important. In the foreword to the first edition of this book, Billy Trolan, an emergency room physician and medical consultant to adventure racing teams, wrote the following:

> The one factor that continues to amaze me is that individuals and teams will spend vast amounts of money, time, and thought on training, equipment, and travel, but little or no preparation on their feet. Too often the result has been that within a few hours to a few days, all that work has been ruined—ruined because the primary mode of transportation has broken down with blisters. This problem is universal with hikers, runners, [anybody doing] any activity that requires feet. Most of these problems could easily be avoided with some preventative care. Other foot problems could have been taken care of with early treatment, stopping a small problem from becoming a costly one.

The most important factor is knowing what your feet need and how to do it before you have to do it. I have patched many feet at ultras and adventure races and have found that most racers have a fairly good knowledge base of what they should be doing. They know it's smart to wear the right kind of socks and to have footwear that fits well. Many have also made foot-care kits for their crews. I would guess that about 30 to 40 percent are well versed in what their feet need and how to do it. The other 60 to 70 percent just wing it. They've read about foot care but somehow it falls lower on the priority list than does training, finding foods they can tolerate, locating the right flashlight for night running, and other choices. So they start their race and manage well for a while—until problems develop.

Ultrarunner Gillian Robinson shares a story from one of her long races that illustrates what all athletes need to learn:

> I sat for a shoe change and foot fix-up. I wasn't exactly sure what to do with my feet. I had taped the balls of my feet and my big toes. The big-toe taping wasn't working out so well. On the left, it had rubbed

the next toe to cause a big ugly blister that had to be lanced. On the right, maybe the taping was too tight, because the big toenail was bruised at the base. I put Second Skin on the left toe and taped it up with Micropore tape. For the right toe, I just cut off the existing tape and hoped for the best. I sprayed my feet with Desenex to cool them down and dry them out, and then smeared them all over with Hydropel, which is a lubricant. I changed to new socks and different shoes. I felt a lot better. My toes didn't feel perfect, but better.

To have and keep healthy feet, you have to know what works for them in the sports in which you participate. You also have to know what to do when what worked no longer works—in other words, a fallback plan with the equipment to implement it and the knowledge to use it.

Hard-Won Lessons

- Learn what lubricant works, but have a container of powder handy.
- Learn what socks work, but have one or two extra pairs of other types.
- Learn how to tape your toes, heels, and every other part of your feet just in case blisters form.
- Learn how to tape like a pro, and then practice taping, and then practice some more. Then start over until your taping is perfect.
- Learn how to lance blisters and patch over them.
- Learn what happens to your feet when you don't change wet socks. Your feet become macerated and feel as though one humongous blister is covering the bottom of each foot.
- Learn that something simple like properly trimming and filing your toenails can prevent toe blisters and even black toenails.

The bottom line is that if you don't consciously learn what works for your feet, you will learn the hard way. Prevention is *proactive*. Time spent being proactive in preventing problems will pay off in the long run. Taking a proactive approach will mean you spend less time being *reactive* to problems when you have neither the time to spare nor readily available materials.

The key to making prevention work is to find what works for you in the environment where you will use it. In other words, try the fix in the context in which it will be used. When you are trying to find what works for you on trails, running on roads will not typically provide the same results as actually running on trails. Walking around town wearing a backpack and your hiking boots is not the same as hiking on a rocky trail with uneven terrain. It may help to break in your boots but will not give the same feeling as a rough rocky trail. I made my own gaiters for trail running after determining that the dirt getting into my shoes was causing hot spots and blisters. Getting out on the trails will help you determine whether your footwear fits and if there are problems to correct. That's being proactive.

Mike Palmer has spent years finding what works for his feet: "This can be one hell of a frustrating process—you may have an overwhelming urge to throw in the towel and take up playing chess instead. One runner will swear on his mother's grave that such-and-such a thing solved his problem, but his solution won't work at all for you." It cannot be overstressed; you must find what works for your feet. Taking the time to learn what works for your feet is the key to being proactive.

Cathy Sassin knows what her feet need. One of the United States' top adventure racers, she has trekked across the sands of Utah and South Africa, the volcanoes of Ecuador, and the glaciers of British Columbia and Patagonia. She has bushwhacked through Maine, spelunked through Borneo, paddled and ridden through New Zealand and Australia, and raced across New England.

On the SealSkinz Website, Cathy sums up the method behind her success:

Tried & True Foot Care

The four keys to winning any extreme sport are a strong mental attitude, working as a team rather than as an individual, keeping hydrated, and having a great foot-care regimen. After every race me and my team are generally the only ones without bloody, blistered feet, and everyone wants to know my secret, so here it is!

■ Spray feet with tincture of benzoin spray. This provides a tough protective layer where blisters usually form. Be careful not to apply too much or in the creases of the feet as it will crack and dry the skin.

■ Put a thin layer of Hydropel around the feet over the tincture of benzoin. Hydropel is a Vaseline-like substance that offers some water repellency and a little lubrication without friction.

■ It is essential to keep feet comfortable and dry, so I put on a pair of liner socks (I recommend Wigwam) followed by a pair of SealSkinz waterproof socks. SealSkinz come in a variety of styles, but I recommend either the insulated socks (for colder conditions), over-the-calf socks, or their new WaterBlocker sock with in-cuff seal to keep water out even when feet are submerged! All SealSkinz products feature a patented, state-of-the-art Moisture Vapor Transpiration design and a unique, breathable inner fabric membrane to draw perspiration away from the skin as well as keep water out. Plus, their stretch-to-fit, seamless design helps prevent blisters and chafing even after the most extreme activities.

■ Wear a pair of boots or running shoes that are very lightweight but stable enough to handle rigorous terrain (every ounce counts in racing). When wearing running shoes, choose a lightweight model that allows water to squeeze out as you run.

■ Add a pair of gaiters to further prevent grit, dirt, and small rocks from getting in the boots, which will help prevent unnecessary friction and abrasions.

■ Use a pair of adjustable walking poles (I use Leki poles) to help distribute weight throughout the body every step of the way. Poles are great for balance on the downhills and help feet from taking a pounding.

—Cathy Sassin, globe-trotting adventure racer

Components of Prevention

The one problem with our feet that we experience most often, which drives us crazy and costs us time and, in some cases, leads to unfulfilled dreams, is blisters. Although the following chapters deal with all aspects of foot care, the prevalent theme is keeping our feet healthy by preventing "dreaded" blisters.

Blister prevention requires a combination of components: socks, powders, lubricants, skin tougheners, taping, orthotics, nutrition for the feet, proper hydration, antiperspirants for the feet, gaiters, laces, and frequent sock and shoe changes, among others. You need to start with proper fitting shoes with a quality insole. No matter how well you tape, or how good your socks are, or how good any other component is, if the shoes fit incorrectly, you will have problems. The materials and compounds you apply to your skin (powder, lubricant, or tape) must work together with anything surrounding your feet (the insoles, orthotics, socks, shoes, gaiters, and even your shoelaces) in order to prevent blisters. Cutting corners on any one of the factors can increase the chances of blisters.

Imagine a triangle with heat, friction, and moisture at its three sides. These three factors combine to make the skin more susceptible to blisters. Dr. David Hannaford, a podiatrist and runner, stresses, "If you eliminate any one of the three factors, you eliminate the blister."

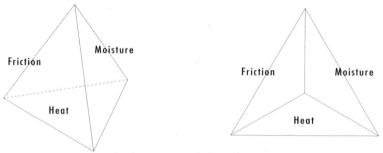

The three causes of blister formation.

Imagine that this triangle sits on a base that has two levels. Each level of the base is a circle made up of components that can prevent these three conditions from forming. Closest to the triangle is the upper circle of socks, powders, and lubricants—the first line of defense against blisters. Friction, which produces heat, can be reduced by wearing a sock with wicking properties or by using foot powders or lubricants. Moisture can also be reduced by wearing socks with wicking properties and by using powders.

Socks come in either single- or double-layer construction. Some single-layer socks, particularly those without wicking properties, allow friction to develop between the feet and the socks, which in turn can create blisters. Double-layer socks allow the sock layers to move against each other or the two mate-

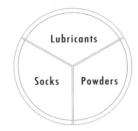

The first level of defense against blisters.

rials to work together, which reduces friction between the feet and the socks.

Powders reduce friction by reducing moisture on the skin that in turn reduces friction between the feet and the socks.

Lubricants create a shield to protect skin that is in contact with skin and socks during motion. This lubricant shield reduces chafing, which in turn reduces friction.

Now, imagine another underlying circle made up of components that play a strong supporting role in prevention—the second level of defense against blisters. This lower circle is made up of skin tougheners, taping, orthotics, nutrition for the feet and proper hydration, antiperspirants for the feet, gaiters, lacing, and frequent sock and shoe changes. Each can contribute to the prevention of blisters and other problems. You could argue that these outer components should be identified as major components, and to some extent you may be right. Some components may be more important for your feet than for mine. The trick is to determine what we each need to keep our feet healthy under the stresses of our particular sport.

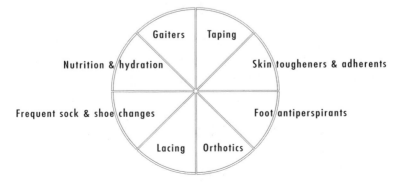

The second level of defense against blisters.

Skin tougheners form a coating to protect and toughen the skin. These products also help tape and blister patches adhere better to the skin.

Taping provides a barrier between the skin and socks so friction is reduced. Proper taping adds an extra layer of skin (the tape) to the foot to prevent hot spots and blisters. Taping can also be a treatment if hot spots and blisters develop. An alternative to taping, ENGO Performance Patches go on the inside your shoe or on your insole. These thin fabric-film composite patches can greatly reduce friction in targeted locations within your footwear by giving a slick, slippery surface to the area of your footwear or insole where friction is a problem. Jelly Toes are silicon gel devices that go over the toes and reduce friction.

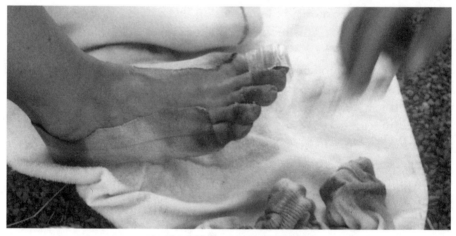

Taping can make the difference between finishing a race and limping your way through (or dropping out).

Orthotics help maintain the foot in a functionally neutral position so arch and pressure problems are relieved. Small pads for the feet may also help correct foot imbalances and pressure points.

Skin care for the feet includes creams and lotions so dry and callused feet are softened. They result in softer and smoother skin. Proper hydration can help reduce swelling of the feet so the occurrence of hot spots and blisters is reduced.

Antiperspirants for the feet help those with excessively sweaty feet by reducing the moisture that makes the feet more prone to blisters.

Gaiters provide protection against dirt, rocks, and grit. These irritants cause friction and blisters as shoes and socks become dirty. Shoe and boot-laces often cause friction or pressure problems. Adjusting laces can relieve this friction and pressure and make footwear more comfortable.

Frequent sock changes help keep the feet in good condition. Wet or moist socks can cause problems. Changing the socks also gives opportunity to reapply either powder or lubricant and deal with any hot spots before they become blisters. Sometimes shoes are also changed as they become overly dirty or wet.

Finding the Right Combination

Each runner and hiker needs to find a prevention strategy that works for him or her. One may use Vaseline, another may use Zeasorb powder, and yet another may pretape his feet. They each may use one of many types and styles of socks. There are many combinations.

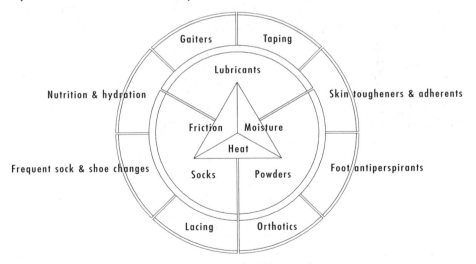

The blister triangle and the two bases of blister-reducing components.

Ultrarunner Dave Scott claims his feet are often "as soft as a baby's bottom" after the 100-mile Western States Endurance Run. Dave has found that he rarely gets foot problems. He trims his toenails, uses a small amount of

Vaseline, and regularly changes his shoes and socks. That is what works for him. At the other extreme is the runner who has the skin falling off his feet from midsoles to heels. One hiker may end a six-day hike having had a few simple foot problems, while another may have suffered with major problems the whole trip—even if they wear the same shoes and socks. Determine what foot problems you normally experience, study this book, and then begin the task of finding what works best for your feet.

Ultrarunner Tim Twietmeyer has won the grueling 100-mile Western States Endurance Run five times while accumulating 22 silver belt buckles for sub-24 hour finishes. Over the past years, in addition to running ultras, he has enjoyed fastpacking in the California High Sierra. He has found the differences interesting.

A week before running a 100-mile trail ultra, Tim trims his toenails as short as possible. The morning of the run he coats his feet with lanolin to reduce friction, provide warmth if running in snow or through water, and make his skin more resilient to getting all wrinkled. Then he pulls on a pair of Thorlo Ultrathin socks. His strategy is "that the more sock you wear, the more moisture close to the foot. The more moisture, the more blisters and skin problems." He usually wears the same pair of shoes and socks the entire way. Tim acknowledges "my feet don't usually have problems, and when they do, I'm close enough to the end to gut it out."

Tim has found that fastpacking affects his feet differently. When he hiked the John Muir Trail in 1992 (doing 210 miles in 5 days and 10 hours), his feet were trashed more than ever before. His group of five experienced ultrarunners averaged 14 hours per day on the rough trail. Tim remembers "we covered the ground so fast that my feet swelled and I almost couldn't get my shoes on the last day." He used the same strategy of using lanolin and thin socks. Instead of running shoes, he chose lightweight hiking boots. Foot repair became the group's daily ritual as the 40-mile days took their toll. They realized that "an important strategy for keeping our feet from getting any worse was to get that first piece of duct tape on in just the right spot and make it stick. If we did that, our feet held up pretty well." By the end of the fifth day, the last piece of duct tape had been used on their feet. Tim's cardinal rule for fastpacking is "Keep your feet dry." That can be hard to do when fighting afternoon thunderstorms, but when your feet are wet too long, it's only a matter of time before they blister. Whether running ultras or fastpacking, Tim knows the importance of keeping his feet healthy, and he has experimented to find what works well for him.

We need to understand the importance of other elements that contribute to prevention. Proper strength training and conditioning will help make the foot and ankle stronger and more resistant to sprains and strains. Good care of the skin will help prevent calluses. Quality insoles and orthotics can help prevent or relieve the problems of plantar fasciitis, Achilles tendinitis, heel pain, metatarsalgia, Morton's neuroma, Morton's foot, sesamoiditis, corns, and bunions. Good-fitting footwear will help prevent problems with toe-nails, arches, and blisters. In short, everything you put on or around your foot becomes related to how well your foot functions.

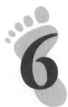

Socks

Socks perform four basic functions: cushioning, protection, warmth, and absorption of moisture off the skin. The sock fabric and weave will determine how well they do each. Socks made from synthetic fabrics wick moisture away from the skin and through the sock to its outer surface where it can evaporate.

Although I usually inform athletes of their foot-care options and advise them to make the best choices for them, I have two absolutes. The first deals with socks. Serious athletes should avoid 100-percent cotton socks like the plague and always use moisture-wicking socks. The second absolute is covered in the chapter on gaiters (see page 129). And yet some athletes prefer common cotton crew socks, and others swear by synthetic socks or synthetic double-layer socks. If cotton crew socks work for you, continue using them. If, however, hot spots and/or blisters plague you, consider trying other types of socks. Some have discovered socks with individual toes and like these because they avoid dirt and grime collecting between the toes and causing friction.

For my first 24-hour track run, I wore thick cotton socks and used gobs of Vaseline on my feet. That was what everyone else seemed to be doing, so that was what I did. It didn't take long for blisters that reduced me to a slow walk to develop on my heels and toes. Even so, I managed to get in a respectable 103 miles. Without the early foot problems, I am sure I could have done another 10 miles. I learned the hard way what did not work on my feet and set out to find what did work.

Not everyone needs a primer on how to put on your socks, but it is important to know a few tricks. Although it seems like a simple thing, it can make the difference between sore, blistered feet and happy feet.

Mindfulness: The Art of Putting on Your Socks

First be sure your socks are clean and free of debris. Hold them by the cuff, pull them through the closed fist of the other hand, and then whip them in the air a couple times. Turn them inside out and then repeat. If the socks have a heavy seam at the toe, wear them inside out. Next massage your feet and between the toes making sure there is absolutely no grit or other debris. Then either roll or bunch the socks up so the toes can be placed in the toe of the sock. Be sure the seam is across the top of the toes and if possible not lapping around the small toe. Now bring the sock up over the rest of the foot and up the leg, use a massaging motion to be sure there are no wrinkles and to detect any rough spots or debris.

Next, remove the insert from your shoe and inspect it. Remove any lint, toe jam, or other debris. Now bang the shoes together sole to sole a couple times and then tap the heel on the ground. Now shake out any debris and reach inside and feel all surfaces for debris or other problems. Replace the inserts and put on your shoes. Sounds complicated but the whole process takes less than a minute and can prevent many foot problems.

—Rick Schick, ultrarunner & physician's assistant

Clean socks can feel heavenly. When hiking, wash yesterday's socks and let them dry on the back of your pack. Try to change socks several times during a 100-mile run and once during a 50-mile run. During multi-day events, try to change socks several times a day. If clean socks are unavailable from your crew, try to wash the dirty socks so they are clean for later use.

You may be one of a growing number of athletes who wear socks inside out. Rob Langsdorf recommends simply turning your socks inside out to help prevent blisters: "Most socks have a rib near the toe where the sock is pulled together. The manufacturers put this on the inside of the sock, so it looks nice. Unfortunately it tends to rub the tops and sides of the toes and can cause blisters."

At summer's end, the usefulness of many of your shoes and socks may also be coming to an end. Go through your drawers and pull out all your socks. Put your hand inside and check for threadbare areas under the heels and forefoot and for holes in the toes. If you find these, toss the socks and go shopping for new ones—being sure to get socks with moisture-wicking fabrics.

Sock Fibers & Construction

Socks come in a variety of fabrics: cotton, cotton blends, synthetics, silk, wool and wool blends, and fleece. An overview of these materials provides insights into their uses. Read the product information on the sock's packaging and try several types to find those that work best for you.

Natural, Synthetic & Combination Materials

COTTON socks provide no wicking or insulating properties, and therefore moisture is retained against the skin. In damp or wet cotton, your feet are generally wet, cold, and more prone to blistering. Do yourself a favor and avoid 100-percent cotton socks.

COTTON BLENDS containing Lycra, nylon, rayon, and acrylic offer a limited advantage over a pure cotton sock.

SYNTHETICS offer protection against blisters caused by moisture, poor fit, hot spots, slippage, and friction. These are made of hydrophobic materials, meaning they don't like moisture or water. Moisture-wicking fabrics such as Capilene, CoolMax, Olefin, and polypropylene wick moisture and perspiration away from the skin to the outer layer of the sock. Synthetic insulators like Hollofil, Thermax, and Thermastat help provide insulation. Some of these socks have a single layer, while others have double layers. Most synthetic socks use one of the above fabrics blended with cotton, nylon, Lycra spandex, or acrylic.

SILK socks are slick and are generally used as liners. Offering low wicking properties and low heat retention, they do not dry as fast as the newer synthetics.

WOOL wicks while retaining its cushioning but can be scratchy and rough.

WOOL BLENDS are comfortably warm in winter and cool in summer. Socks made from worsted wool are soft and durable. Merino wool, from sheep with a lighter and softer coat, is less resilient but very soft and comfortable. Wool may also be blended with other fabrics.

FLEECE socks are soft, provide exceptional warmth, and dry faster than wool.

The weave of the sock will vary depending on the material. Socks will range from a loose weave to a dense weave. A loose weave feels coarse and provides less insulation. A dense weave feels softer and generally offers more cushioning. Put your hand inside a sock and stretch the foot portion with your fingers to see the weave. Denser-weave socks will show less space between the fibers.

Double-layer socks can help reduce or eliminate blisters. The two layers moving against each other instead of against the skin reduces skin friction. Most double-layer socks utilize wicking properties to move moisture away from the feet. Before wearing any double-layer sock, align the layers with your hand and then roll the socks onto the foot for the best fit.

Technology is moving faster than we can keep up—even in socks. Injinji makes toe socks with a four-point anatomical molding system. These Tetrasoks are constructed without seams. With individual toes to protect each toe, they help those prone to toe blisters. Made with CoolMax, nylon, and spandex, they conform to the shape of your feet.

Wigwam has introduced a new InGenius Dry-Lined Comfort sock that knits a liner sock and outer sock into one piece of fabric. The inner liner side of the sock wicks, while the outer layer is merino wool. The blend of the two makes for a sock that will keep your feet comfortable, dry, and more blister free.

Oxysocks cover the calf and stimulate circulation in the muscles, providing support and enhancing stamina. By applying graduated pressure to the lower extremities, starting at the foot and up to the calf, blood is returned more rapidly to the heart and lungs. The patented technology shows a quicker return of oxygenated blood to the legs and reduces fatigue.

Outlast Technologies has pioneered the development of phase change materials that absorb, store, and release energy in response to body heat. The result is Outlast's patented Adaptive Comfort technology, producing a range of smart textiles that respond to the wearer's body temperature as he or she moves between various indoor and outdoor climates. This technology is being added to socks and insoles.

Blister Guard technology utilizes Teflon as a low-friction fiber that prevent hot spots that cause blisters, abrasions, and calluses. The Teflon fibers are woven into the fabric of the sock at the toes, forefoot, and the heels. These socks have undergone strenuous tests, achieving an 80 to 100 percent reduction of blisters, and they are being marketed by various sock companies with combinations of traditional fibers such as acrylic, wool, nylon, and polyester, as well as performance fibers such as CoolMax and Lycra. John Prohira recalls that he "thought that blisters were a fact of life or dues to be paid." Then he was given a pair of Blister Guard socks by a friend and wore them on an 11-hour run with no hot spots or blisters. Look for the Blister Guard symbol.

Asics has introduced the Kayano sock that has anatomically correct right and left foot construction. And Fox River has a line of socks called Fox River for Women. These socks have a more rounded toe and flex-stretch heels designed for a woman's feet.

Buying Socks

Buy socks that fit your feet. The heels, toes, and length should fit snugly without sagging or being stretched too tight. Socks that are too big will bunch up and cause friction and skin irritation. Socks that are too small can cause the toes and joints to rub harder against the socks. Turn the socks inside out and look at the toe seams. Avoid those with bulky seams because they can rub, causing hot spots and blisters. After buying socks be sure to try them on with your shoes or boots to be sure they fit together and are not too tight. Remember also to discard socks when they become threadbare and too thin to provide their advertised benefits. The heels of your socks are a good indication of the amount of padding and loft.

Many stores offer a basket of socks to use when trying on shoes and boots. Avoid these if possible, and instead use your own socks when shopping. This way you will get to feel the fit with your personal socks and avoid picking up a foot fungus from another shopper.

TIP: Go for the Garter

Sock garters can prevent socks from slipping and getting wrinkled inside of the shoe, which can lead to blisters and hot spots. This is especially true when feet are wet either from rain, stream crossings, or excessive perspiration. It also is more of a problem on trails with steep climbs and descents, although it can also happen when hiking on dry, level surfaces. Making a sock garter can help to prevent the problem.

Go to a craft store or sewing supply center and buy a couple feet of 1¼ inch-width elastic, the kind used in clothing. Be sure to get the ribbed or "roll proof" variety. Measure around your leg at the narrowest point, just above the ankle, and then make a loop of the elastic about one half inch shorter. When placed over the sock at that point, the garter should feel snug but not tight.

Sock designs and the sock market change so fast that company Websites are often the best source of information for specific lines of socks. Each company introduces new versions of their socks each year. As an example, one sock company brochure offers four types of sandal socks, nine types of running/walking socks, twelve types of hiking socks, and the list goes on. New fabrics and combinations of fabrics make the sock selection ever changing. Your local stores will have displays of many of these socks or check out the Websites listed below (and there are many more sock manufacturers out there). Investigate your sock options and talk to others about their preferences to determine which socks may be best for your hiking needs.

If you have a hard time finding the socks you want, you might check out **www.justsocks.com** or **www.thesockcompany.com**.

Specialty Socks

The following sections identify specific socks for running, hiking, and sandals, and others cover sock liners and high-technology oversocks. Many of these socks may be used for running, hiking, and adventure racing. Check them out at a store near you to feel them and read their packaging information. The products listing at the end of this chapter notes which companies make socks for each type of sport.

Running Socks

The following companies offer excellent running sock choices: BaySix, Bridgedale, Defeet, Fox River, Goldtoe Gear, InGenius, Injinji, Oxysocks, Powersox, Seamless Socks, The Sock Guy, SmartWool, Thorlo, Wigwam, and Wrightsock.

Hiking Socks

Hiking socks are different from running socks. Hikers most often wear crew or high-top socks. Some wear a wool outer sock with a liner that has wicking properties. Hikers could also try the thinner double-layer wicking socks in a crew style. These wear well, wick moisture away, and are made to reduce the possibility of blisters.

Pacific Crest Trail hiker Matthew Jankowicz used to get blisters, especially on long hikes over 20 miles a day. He tried tape, moleskin, and different kinds of boots. Finally, he switched to wearing three pairs of socks and it worked. He uses one pair of wicking socks over which he wears two pair of boot socks. Matthew says, "I know some people think I'm crazy, but it works very well for me and I have hiked thousands of miles this way without getting any blisters on my feet."

Another hiker, going by the trail name of Morning Glory, found that wearing a thin liner sock, a Thorlo sock, and finally a wool-blend hiking sock worked well. She bought boots with enough room to accommodate the three pairs of socks. When wearing heavy socks for winter or otherwise, wear a boot a half size larger than normal. If you wear your normal size boot, it compresses the heavy sock and at best you gain little in the way of insulation. In the worst case, it is so tight it inhibits blood flow to the toes and results in frostbite.

The following companies offer good-quality socks: Acorn Fleece Socks, Bridgedale, Dahlgren, Fox River, Goldtoe Gear, Injinji, Patagonia, REI Socks, SmartWool, Thermohair Socks, Thorlo, Wigwam, and Wyoming Wear.

Sock Liners

Sock liners are thin and smooth, and they are usually worn under a heavier insulating or cushioning sock, typically wool. They are lightweight and quick drying. Most liners are made from hydrophobic fibers to wick moisture away from the foot and into the outer sock. A liner will perform in tandem with the outer sock the same way as double-layer socks; friction will occur between the two layers and not against the skin, reducing the chance of blisters. When shopping for liners, look for a style with wicking properties. While many runners are converting to the double-layer socks, some still prefer a two-sock system using liners.

Some athletes like ankle-high nylons as an inner sock! Sid Snyder found that by wearing ankle high nylons under his Thorlo socks, he does not get blisters. No tape and no Vaseline—just the nylons. He had blistered so badly on another long trail event that he was on crutches for three days and knew he had to try something new. Be sure to try this combination before a competitive event. Try them with the sock you normally wear, preferably a wicking sock. When using nylons for trail running or hiking, be sure to try them on uphills and downhills since some individuals may be bothered by the slippery smooth nylon. You may want to test various styles of nylons—some are more slippery than others.

The following companies offer good-quality sock liners: Fox River, Helly-Hansen Polypro Liners, SmartWool, and Wigwam.

High-Technology Oversocks

Oversocks are special high-technology socks that combine waterproof technology and the comfort of traditional socks into a somewhat baggy-looking sock. They were developed for anyone who participates in outdoor activities during which feet are exposed to water. They keep feet dry and comfortable even though the shoes or boots may be soaked and muddy. Widely used by hunters and fishermen, they are being discovered by runners, hikers, and adventure racers.

National champion ultrarunner Roy Pirrung tested the high-technology oversock SealSkinz for a year in all kinds of weather. Roy recalls his win at the 100K Glacial Trail Run, a grueling race through the wet Kettle Moraine State Forest in Wisconsin: "It had rained the day before and conditions were sloppy. As other runners stopped every 10 miles to change their wet socks, I just raced ahead. I ended up finishing the race within 25 seconds of the course record and without any blisters." In wet and cold conditions, over-socks can work wonders. Roy found that SealSkinz have helped him to train outside in minus 25-degree weather with a windchill factor of minus 80. His feet "stayed warm, dry, and comfortable."

SealSkinz Socks are seamless waterproof socks that use moisture vapor transpiration (MVT) technology. The socks are made in a thin, lightweight, three-layer design. An inner CoolMax liner wicks moisture away from the skin while a middle layer of vapor-permeable membrane allows perspiration to escape and prevents water from entering. The outer layer uses nylon for abrasion resistance and durability. Their seamless design gives them a positive edge in preventing blisters. Their WaterBlocker socks are fully immersible and their revolutionary in-cuff seal ensures a tight, waterproof fit to keep out everything from water to grit. All-Season socks have a Lycra spandex cuff to ensure the socks will stay up, but the cuff will allow water in. An over-the-calf sock is also available. A new ChillBlocker sock made to protect feet from extreme temperatures will have a Polartec fleece liner.

Many adventure racers use SealSkinz socks to keep their feet free of blisters, abrasions caused by dirt and grime, and the effects of water immersion during their long, multiday competition. Adventure racer Rebecca Rusch was on Team Montrail at the Primal Quest Adventure race in Telluride, Colorado, where the team used SealSkinz to help them to a second-place finish. Rebecca says, "The only thing I've found for keeping out grit, sand, (and leeches) are SealSkinz socks. I've used them in Borneo, Philippines, and Vietnam, and I will use them in Fiji. They're hot in these environments but keep your feet clean and healthy."

Rocky Gore-Tex Oversocks from REI are waterproof, breathable, and designed to be worn over a pair of thin wicking socks. The socks have a Gore-Tex membrane laminated between inner and outer fabric layers. The inner seams are sealed with Gore-Seam tape. The sole and bottom panel are made of a nonstretch Gore-Tex fabric to increase durability and prevent slippage. The upper panels are stretchable Gore-Tex fabric for flexibility and conformity to the foot's shape. A spandex cuff helps the socks stay up. When wearing these socks, watch for skin irritations caused by the inner seams.

TIP: New Life for Old Bags

An alternative to these type socks is to put on a pair of thick socks and then a soft plastic bag over the feet, finally adding a thin outer sock. The inner socks, in the plastic bags, will get damp from body sweat and heat, but will stay reasonably comfortable compared to totally wet feet. The plastic bags that bread or newspapers come in work well, but check them first for leaks by blowing in them and squeezing them lightly while holding them closed.

Seirus Neo-Sock and StormSocks rely on closed-cell insulation to provide warmth for winter activities. They are made from four-way stretch neoprene with breathable macro-porous technology to prevent moisture buildup while sealing in body heat. These socks have a nylon fabric on either side of the neoprene that allows moisture to pass through. The StormSock has an outer layer of Lycra, an inner membrane of high-technology Weather Shield that stops wind and water, and it is lined with Polartec fleece. Both socks have seams that should be checked for waterproofing.

For more information about Rocky Gore-Tex Oversocks, SealSkinz Socks, and Seirus Neo Sock and Stormsocks, see the product listing at the end of this chapter.

Try any type of oversocks before a competitive event. You may find they do not work on your feet. Some athletes roll the tops down when not going through water to ventilate the feet. Oversocks work best when used with a CoolMax or other wicking-material sock liner. This further enhances moisture dispersion as well as comfort. Care must be taken when pulling the socks on or off to avoid tearing the inner membrane. A torn membrane will allow water to penetrate at the tear site.

Unless you are wearing the SealSkinz WaterBlocker socks, your oversocks should not be submersed in water over the cuffs. If the cuff is loose fitting, water may get inside. Once water has gone down the leg into the sock, the wicking process slows or stops, depending on the amount of water in the sock. Over time, the body's heat combined with the wicking action of the CoolMax liner may dry the inside of the socks, but this depends on both the amount of water inside the sock and the degree of activity. Roy Pirrung recommends wearing tights over the cuffs to provide a covering seal.

The Option of Not Wearing Socks

In 1973 a running magazine advertised "New, lean, and luxurious—the first sockless athletic shoe." After three years of development, Bare Foot Gear offered the "Original Sockless Shoe" with prime leather inside and out, no staples or nails, no seams or ridges, and no textiles to touch your foot, just unpainted and unsealed leather. Cupping the foot only at the heel and instep, it offered a large space up front for flexion and good air circulation. It claimed that with a drier foot, friction is minimized. Looking at the ad today, we might find humor in the ad's claim that "Most men prefer no socks because of the sheer maleness of the feel."

Some people—male and female—prefer not to wear socks. Matt Mahoney found that for him, the best way to prevent blisters was to train for them. Walking barefoot and sometimes running barefoot on grass, dirt, or sand toughened the skin on his feet. He does not wear socks with shoes but rotates between several brands of shoes to develop calluses at every spot that could rub. Matt found that socks caused his feet to slide around inside his shoes, and he couldn't grip the trail on steep hills. When he finds spots rubbing, he uses tape, Vaseline, or a blister pad.

This type of barefoot running or running in shoes without socks takes time and careful monitoring of your feet to avoid problems. Matt has conditioned his feet by walking a mile barefoot on roads every day. He estimates he runs 15 percent of the time barefoot on grass and dirt and the other 85 percent in shoes without socks. He has strengthened the small muscles and tendons in his feet. The skin on the bottom of his feet has toughened to provide some degree of protection for running barefoot. Gradually toughen your feet with short periods of barefoot walking before trying to run barefoot. If trying to go without socks, check your shoes for rough seams or ridges that can cut into your feet. Like Matt, use tape or a lubricant on areas that rub. Matt strongly believes we need to "learn to run in simple shoes, sandals, or barefoot as people have done for thousands of years before Nike." Barefoot running and hiking is becoming more accepted.

When venturing barefoot onto trails or even pavement, you should take a few precautions. Start slowly with short barefoot excursions to give your feet time to adjust. Your feet are used to the support and cushioning of shoes, and going without will make a sudden change. Be attentive to the conditions of the path underfoot. Your feet can be cut or punctured by debris on the road or trail. If you want to run barefoot, start by walking. This strengthens the skin, muscles, tendons, and ligaments of the feet and ankles.

Walking and running barefoot can be an excellent way to condition your feet in order to prevent blisters when you do wear boots or shoes. Your skin will be tougher and you may develop calluses. Yet, be forewarned—this is no guarantee that you will not get blisters! Kevin Sayers had feet that were a "bushman/firewalker's dream, impervious to almost all minor punctures and discomfort." Yet he would get blisters underneath his calluses on the balls of his feet. He learned that he would rather tape a blister that he could see rather than one that's beneath the skin. Blisters under skin-toughened calluses can take four to six weeks to heal, significantly longer than the usual two weeks it takes a normal blister to heal.

Lest you think that going barefoot is only for walking and runners, consider the group Barefoot Hikers. Barefoot Chris (his trail name), a member of Barefoot Hikers, recalls the shocked reaction of hikers they encountered while on a weeklong barefoot backpacking trip on the Appalachian Trail. They heard stories of many other barefoot hikers, including at least two that had done the entire trail without shoes. Those interested in exploring the outdoors barefoot should check out Running Barefoot (**www.runningbarefoot.org**) and the Society for Barefoot Living (**www.barefooters.org**). The book *The Barefoot Hiker* by Richard Frazine is about hiking barefoot.

SOCK PRODUCTS

ACORN FLEECE SOCKS (hiking socks), **Acorn,**
(800) **USA-CORN, www.acornearth.com**

BAYSIX (running socks),
(888) **BAY-SIX1, www.BaySixUSA.com**

BRIDGEDALE (running, hiking socks),
(888) **79-SOCKS, www.bridgedaleusa.com**

DAHLGREN (hiking socks), **Dahlgren Footwear Inc.,**
(800) **635-8539, www.dahlgrenfootwear.com**

DEFEET (running socks), **Defeet International,**
(800) **688-3067, www.defeet.com**

FOX RIVER (running, hiking & liner socks),
(888) **288-2431, www.foxsox.com**

GOLDTOE GEAR (running, hiking socks),
(336) **229-3700, www.goldtoegear.com**

HELLY-HANSEN POLYPRO LINERS (liner socks), **Patagonia,**
(800) **336-9090**

INGENIUS (running, hiking socks), **Wigwam Mills Inc.,**
(800) **558-7760, www.ingeniussocks.com**

INJINJI (running, hiking socks), **Injinji Footwear,**
(888) **465-4654, www.injinji.com**

OXYSOCKS (running socks),
(887) **669-9769, www.oxysox.com**

PATAGONIA (hiking socks),
(800) **336-9090, www.patagonia.com**

SOCK PRODUCTS

POWERSOX (running socks), **www.moretzsports.com**

REI SOCKS (hiking socks),
(800) 426-4840, www.rei.com

ROCKY GORE-TEX OVERSOCKS (oversocks), **REI,**
(800) 426-4840, www.rei.com

SEALSKINZ SOCKS (oversocks), **Danalco,**
(800) 216-9938, www.danalco.com

SEAMLESS SOCKS (running socks), **SmartKnitACTIVE,**
(888) 466-0001, www.smartknitactive.com

SEIRUS NEO-SOCK & STORMSOCKS (oversocks), **Seirus Innovative**
Accessories, (800) 447-3787, www.serius.com

SMARTWOOL (running, hiking, liner socks),
(800) 550-9665, www.smartwool.com

THE SOCK GUY (running socks),
(888) 232-5376, www.sockguy.com

THERMOHAIR SOCKS (hiking socks), **Thermohair (Canada),**
(877) 766-4247, www.thermohair.com

THORLO (running, hiking socks),
(800) 438-0286, www.thorlo.com

WIGWAM (running, hiking, liner socks), **Wigwam Mills Inc.**
(800) 558-7760, www.wigwam.com

WRIGHTSOCK (running socks), **(800) 654-7191**

WYOMING WEAR (hiking socks),
(800) WYO-WEAR, www.wyomingwear.com

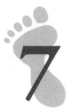

Compounds for the Feet

Then here are three compounds you can put on your feet. Some athletes will use only one, while others may use two, or at times, all three. The most commonly applied compound is lubricant, typically used to make the feet slippery to reduce friction. Powder is used more and more frequently as athletes learn how dry feet are subject to far less friction. A small percentage of athletes use an antiperspirant to control excessive sweating of their feet.

Powders

One of the best ways of preventing hot spots and blisters is by using either powder or a lubricant on your feet. Both work well, but one may be better suited to your feet. If you have been using a lubricant on your feet and still get blisters, first try one of the newer "state-of-the-art" lubricants. If the blisters continue, try powder. Some skin will respond better to being dry, and powders that prevent moisture buildup on the skin are a good choice. For other athletes, lubricants are a better choice. If you have continued problems, try several of each.

Using Powder

There are powders and then there are powders. Cornstarch and talcum powder have been used for years as foot powders, but times and powders

P O W D E R   P R O D U C T S

BLISTERSHIELD MIRACLE POWDER made by Two Toms helps prevent hot spots, blisters, and calluses. Containing micronized wax and cornstarch, the very slick powder reduces friction and heat buildup. BlisterShield repels water by allowing vapor (perspiration) to pass through it and keeps moisture off your skin. **Two Toms, (603) 924-7847, www.twotomsllc.com**

BROMI-TALC is made by Gordon Laboratories as a triple-action foot powder containing potassium alum, an astringent that retards perspiration, and bentonite, an absorption agent that absorbs 18 times its own weight in moisture. Bromi-Talc Plus powder contains additional properties to control excessive foot odor. Both powders are available only by special order through your local drugstore, pharmacy, or podiatrist. **Gordon Laboratories, (800) 356-7870**

CORNSTARCH is an inexpensive powder that can be found at your local supermarket. It works as an absorbent and can be used on feet.

GOLD BOND is a medicated body powder that contains active ingredient zinc oxide as a skin protector and menthol to cool and relieve itching. Use the extra-strength powder for maximum benefits in absorbing excessive moisture. Gold Bond can be found in your local drugstore and pharmacy.

ODOR-EATER'S FOOT POWDER is 25 times more absorbent than talc and also destroys foot odor. It can be found in most drugstores and pharmacies.

ZEASORB is a super-absorbent powder, which absorbs six times its weight in moisture—four times more than plain talcum powder. Zeasorb contains talc, a highly absorbent polymer-carbohydrate acrylic copolymer, and microporous cellulose. This powder is very efficient and works without caking. The talc provides softness and lubrication to reduce friction and heat buildup. Zeasorb-AF (which contains 2 percent miconazole nitrate) provides broad antifungal therapy and moisture control. Zeasorb-AF Lotion/Powder is a unique product for patients who need an antifungal lotion. It offers the ease of lotion application, and then uniquely transforms into a powder, leaving a cool, soft, powdery feeling on the skin, a process that reduces the risk of powder inhalation. Zeasorb is made by Stiefel Laboratories and can be found in your local drug store or pharmacy.

have changed. Having tried a super-absorbent powder, I would never again use a plain powder. Powders can be effective in reducing moisture on the feet, which in turn reduces friction and prevents blisters. Their effectiveness depends on their ability to absorb moisture while not caking into clumps, which can cause skin irritations and blisters. When using powders, remember to reapply the powder at regular intervals or after the feet have been exposed to water. If you have problems with athlete's foot or other skin problems, use an antifungal medicated powder.

After lightly powdering your feet, massage the powder between the toes. Then roll your socks on to the level of the heel and put some powder in the socks. Then squeeze off the top of the sock and shake your foot and repeatedly shake the sock until powder comes through the sock.

Athletes who find their feet become too soft and tender with lubricants can use powders as an alternative foot treatment. Hiker and ultrarunner Randy Gehrke tried powders with great success. He regularly powders his feet and changes his socks in 100-mile runs. In his last two 100-mile trail runs, he has not had any problem with his feet.

Lubricants

As with powders, there are lubricants and then there are lubricants. Two of the old-time tried-and-true lubricants are lanolin and Vaseline. However, technology has led to new formulas. Many runners have discovered Bag Balm or Udder Balm, while many adventure racers prefer Hydropel. Others athletes make their own special formulas.

Ultrarunner Robert Boeder used Andrew Lovy's formula (see below) on his feet in 1994 when he completed the Grand Slam of trail ultrarunning, running four 100-mile runs in 14 weeks. Robert comments that "the idea is that these lotional charms will have the desired magical effect and blisters will not arise from my feet during the race."[11] This formula worked well for him. Since that time he switched to Bag Balm and then back to Vaseline, mainly because of its availability. Ultrarunner Jim Benike found success using Udder Balm on his feet and then wearing socks to bed. He used Udder Balm more as a skin softener and conditioner than as a lubricant. Udder creams may go by different names (for example, Bag Balm, Udder Balm, Dr. Naylor's Udder Balm, and Aunt Irma's Udder Balm).

Newer lubricants are being developed that utilize state-of-the-art ingredients to make them more effective. Hydropel contains 30 percent silicone and works effectively to repel moisture away from the skin. ARGear.com's Michael Johnson, an adventure racer, reports on his Website that "Hydropel seems to also protect your feet from water. I don't get soft waterlogged skin on my feet when using it." Using Hydropel or a similar product can help prevent macerated skin so common to feet wet for long periods of time.

Studies have shown that lubricants may initially reduce friction, but over long periods of time they may actually increase it. After one hour the friction levels returned to their baseline factor, and after three hours the friction levels were 35 percent above the baseline. As the lubricants are absorbed into the skin and into the socks, friction returns and increases.[12] Based on this study, we should learn to reapply lubricants at frequent intervals.

Use lubricants on your feet, hands, underarms, inner thighs, and nipples—anywhere you chafe. The important thing to remember about lubricants is to clean off the old coating before applying the new one. This is especially true during trail runs and hiking when dust and dirt buildup can foul the lubricant with grit. Wipe off the old stuff with a cleansing towelette or an alcohol wipe.

As always, try any new product before using it in a competitive event or taking it on a long hike. It is foolhardy to buy something and count on it in competition or on a six-day hike without trying it first. It may not work for you. Try any lubricant on a small patch of skin to be sure you are not allergic to the ingredients.

LUBRICANT PRODUCTS

ANDREW LOVY'S FORMULA was developed over several years and described in an article "New Blister Formula Revealed! Free!"[13] It helped him solve his blister and friction problems. Take Vitamin A and D Ointment, Vaseline, and Desitin ointment, and mix together equal amounts. To this add vitamin E cream and aloe vera cream (the thickness can be varied by the amount of these two ingredients). The result is a salve. For a thinner mixture, use vitamin E and aloe vera ointments instead of the creams. Andrew recommends that the evening before your run, apply a thin layer to clean skin where friction occurs. In the morning, before you run, apply a more generous amount to friction areas. Add more to problem areas as necessary during the run. Shop around to find the ingredients in sizes appropriate for the total amount you want to mix.

AQUAPHOR HEALING OINTMENT is a petroleum-based ointment that can be used as a lubricant on the feet and other body parts. As a healing ointment, Aquaphor can be used after events to return your feet to like-new condition. Available in a 1¾-ounce tube, it can be found in most drugstores. **Aquaphor, www.aquaphorhealing.com**

AVON SILICONE GLOVE is a silicone cream for hands, but it works equally well on feet. Its nongreasy and nonsticky formula lubricates and softens while protecting against dryness and irritants. It is available in a handy 1½-ounce tube. **Avon Products, (800) FOR-AVON, www.avon.com**

BAG BALM comes in a green tin that has become familiar to many athletes. Bag Balm is made and advertised for use on cow udders, but it has found acceptance in sports circles. Consisting of a combination of lanolin, petrolatum, 8-hydroxy, and quinoline sulfate, it has proven to have healing properties. It can be used on cracked, callused, or sore skin, or simply as a lubricant for your feet or other body areas. Available in 1- or 10-ounce tins, it is usually found in drugstores, pet stores, feed stores and tack shops, and hardware stores. **The Dairy Association Co., (800) 232-3610, www.bagbalm.com (no online sales)**

BLISTERSHIELD ROLL-ON adds a smooth, thin, invisible coating to the skin that will not rub off. This coating eliminates or greatly minimizes the friction that causes blisters, chafing, and irritation. A silicone-based product, it is nonstaining, nontoxic, and nongreasy, and it can be used daily. Use it anywhere you chafe. **Two Toms, (603) 924-7847, www.twotomsllc.com**

BODYGLIDE is a petroleum-free lubricant that protects against friction and skin irritation. This product comes in a "glide-on" applicator similar to a deodorant stick. BodyGlide is hypoallergenic, waterproof, nonsticky, nongreasy (so it will not clog pores), and long lasting. Its main ingredients are triglycerides, aloe, and vitamin E. Its applicator makes it awkward to use on toes but easy to apply to other areas. It comes in three sizes. **BodyGlide, (888) 263-9454, www.bodyglide.com**

CHRIS KOCH'S SECRET FORMULA is made by an adventure racer. He suggests mixing a container of Vaseline, a tube of antibacterial ointment, and a tube of antifungal cream in a double boiler. Blend the ingredients and put the mixture in a small plastic jar, squeeze tube, or similar container. Chris has used this formula during multiday adventure races with good success. He usually uses it with a thin liner sock and a heavier outer sock.

LUBRICANT PRODUCTS

GURNEY GOO is made by world-class adventure racer Steve Gurney. This goo is waterproof, which keeps your feet dry and free of those prune wrinkles while reducing friction. Upgraded with silicon technology, it still retains the tried-and-true tea-tree antiseptic additive, which is great for preventing infections. Gurney Goo comes in 100- and 300-gram sizes. **Gurney Winnovation, www.GurneyGears.com**

HYDROPEL SPORTS OINTMENT is a maximum-strength skin protectant and lubricant. It is made with 30 percent silicone, petrolatum, dimethicone, and aluminum starch octonyl-succinate. Used by many adventure racers, it repels moisture away from the skin, helping to prevent blisters. It excels at protecting against friction and can be used anywhere on the body, and it is also rated effective as a protectant against poison ivy and poison oak. Hydropel is sold through many adventure-racing Websites and is available in a 2-ounce tube. **Genesis Pharmaceutical, (800) 459-8663, www.hydropel.com**

LANOLIN CREAM contains lanolin hydrous, a natural topical skin emollient that lubricates, protects, and soothes. It can be found in most drugstores or pharmacies.

SKIN LUBE is a lubricating ointment with a high melting point that gives it longer-lasting protection against blisters and chafing than petroleum jelly. Its main ingredients are petrolatum, zinc stearate, and silicone. Colorless and nonstaining, it can be used on any friction-prone area of the body. It can be found in sporting-goods stores. **Cramer Products, Inc., (800) 255-6621, www.cramersportsmed.com**

SPORTSLICK, created by a sports physician, is a multipurpose lubricant made for athletes. The gel is easily applied to the toes, feet, inner thighs, underarms, nipples, and lips. SportSlick prevents blisters and chafing with antifriction polymers, silicone, and petrolatum that create a silky feel. It also enriches the skin with vitamin E and C, soybean oil, the antibacterial agent Triclosan, and the antifungal agent Tolnaftate (1 percent). SportSlick is available in two sizes. **SportSlick Products, (800) 646-8448, www.sportslick.com**

UDDER BALM has a lemon fragrance, is nongreasy, and is quickly absorbed by the skin. Similar to Bag Balm, Udder Balm was first made for cow udders. With ingredients including lanolin, aloe vera gel, and vitamins A, D, and E, this cream is ideal for relief from rough and cracked skin, and also for corns, cracked cuticles, and sunburn. Udder Balm is available in 4-ounce tubes, a 1-pound jar, and a huge 4-pound jar. **Udder Balm, (205) 970-0622, www.udderbalm.com**

UN-PETROLEUM JELLY is for those who want a lubricant without petroleum. Made from natural plant oils and waxes, it contains castor oil, coconut oil, PG-3 beeswax, sorbitan tritearate, silica, tocopherol (vitamin E), and natural flavors. It soothes and moisturizes dry skin, prevents chafing and windburn, and is a general-purpose lubricant. Made by Autumn Harp, it is usually found in drugstores and health food stores. **Autumn Harp, (802) 453-4807, www.autumnharp.com**

VASELINE is available in three formulas. The old-time standard is 100 percent pure petroleum jelly. Other formulas include Creamy Vaseline with Vitamin E and anti-bacterial Medicated Vaseline. The medicated formula, in particular, should be helpful for runner's feet, underarms, inner thighs, and nipples. Vaseline is available in most drugstores.

Skin Tougheners & Tape Adherents

Some athletes toughen the skin of their feet to prevent blisters. Often athletes think toughened skin or calluses will always prevent blisters. For some it does. Others have found themselves with blisters under the calluses or toughened skin. These blisters are very difficult to treat. You still must use other blister prevention products like moisture wicking socks, lubricants, or powders.

If you wish to try the skin-toughening approach, begin by spending time walking barefoot on various surfaces. Sandals, worn without socks, can build calluses, but be careful that the calluses do not become too thick or rough. As the skin is irritated through exposure to rough surfaces, it thickens and calluses develop. Remember to keep calluses and roughened skin surfaces smooth by using creams, a pumice stone, or a foot file (see "Skin Care" on page 143 and "Skin Disorders" on page 295).

Tom Gets Tough—Why Shouldn't You?

Tom Crawford's Tea & Betadine Skin Toughener was developed by an ultrarunner who has completed numerous ultras including the challenging Death Valley to Mt. Whitney, both one-way and as an out-and-back run. Tom's method begins with mixing 10 Lipton tea bags and 1 cup of Betadine into a half gallon of water. For one week, dip your feet 20 times over the course of a day, letting them air dry between dips. The second week, add 1 cup of salt to the water, tea, and Betadine mixture. Then for one week, soak your feet for 20 minutes at a time, several times daily. Betadine can be found in drugstores and medical supply stores.

Richard Benyo recalled how he used Tom's method to prepare his feet for the Death Valley 300. "Each night I'd pour the solution into a plastic foot bath and keep my soles and toes in the solution for 15 minutes; then I'd alternately raise one foot out of the brew for three minutes, allowing it to dry, then lower it and bring the other foot out. I'd do that for a half hour. Then I'd let them dry and I'd go to bed with orange soles. When I showered the next morning, it would wash off. But little by little, it made my feet more resistant to blisters."[14] Even with this preparation, Richard sometimes found his feet susceptible to blisters.

SKIN TOUGHENERS & ADHERENTS

CRAMER TUF-SKIN has been used for years by athletic trainers as a taping base. It is ideal for pretaping and skin toughening. Its main ingredients are isopropyl alcohol, isobutane, resin, and benzoin. **Cramer Products, Inc., (800) 255-6621, www.cramersportsmed.com**

MUELLER TUFFNER CLEAR SPRAY is used as a base for athletic taping, but it is also identified as a skin toughener. Its main ingredients are acetone, 1,1,1-trichloroethanem isopropanol, resin, and tincture of benzoin. Look for this product at sporting good stores. **Mueller Sports Medicine, Inc., (800) 356-9522, www.muellersportsmed.com**

NEW-SKIN LIQUID BANDAGE comes in either an antiseptic spray or liquid that is useful as a skin protectant or toughener to prevent hot spots and blisters. It dries rapidly to form a tough protective cover that is antiseptic, flexible, and waterproof, while letting the skin breathe. The 1-ounce size is small and convenient. Clean the skin, spray or coat, and let dry. A second coating may be added for additional protection. Keep toes bent when applying and drying. There is no residue or stickiness. Do not apply to infected or draining sites. It is strong smelling stuff, so use with good ventilation and avoid breathing too deeply. Its main ingredients are pyroxylin solution, acetone ACS, oil of cloves, and 8-hydroxyquinoline. Look for New-Skin at drugstores or online. **Medtech Laboratories Inc., (800) 443-4908, www.medtechinc.com**

RUBBING ALCOHOL has been the preference of renowned walker Colin Fletcher as a skin toughener.[15] Use it on your toes, soles, and heels several times daily. While walking and hiking with sore feet, he recommends almost hourly applications of rubbing alcohol followed by foot powder. Rubbing alcohol is available in drugstores.

TINCTURE OF BENZOIN is available in liquid, swabs, or squeeze vials. Commonly used as a tape or bandage adherent, it is sometimes used as a skin toughener. After applying the tincture, let it dry for about three minutes before applying tape. Tincture of benzoin leaves an orange-brownish color on the skin. Avoid getting the tincture into any cuts, abrasions, or open blisters—it can burn! Usually available in liquid form at drugstores, pharmacies, or medical supply stores. Order swabs or squeeze vials from Medco Sports Medicine. **www.medco-athletics.com**

TUF-FOOT is made from nature's healing balsams and other ingredients. Dr. Andrew Bonn created this unique and original compound in 1935. Made exclusively for feet, either human or animal, Tuf-Foot is guaranteed to toughen soft, tender, or sore feet by working on the tissues. This protects against bruises, blisters, and foot soreness. Recommended use is daily until feet are in good condition and then twice weekly. **Bonaseptic Company, (888) TUF-FOOT, www.tuffoot.com**

You can use several products to toughen your skin or choose the tea and Betadine soak (see page 96). You can also use several of the products as tape adherents to help your choice of tape or moleskin better stick to your feet. Without the adherent, most tapes and blister products will begin to peel off after an hour or two. After applying a blister patch or taping your feet, apply a light coating of powder over any dry sprayed area to counteract the adhesive.

Allow the tincture of benzoin or any sticky tape adherent to dry before applying any tape. Generally three minutes' drying time is sufficient. Wet benzoin is very sticky and slippery. Tape and blister-care products can move around on the foot and fold over on themselves, creating problems. Socks can become stuck to your feet and toes can stick together if you do not allow the benzoin time to dry.

Antiperspirants for the Feet

According to the American Podiatric Medical Association, our feet have approximately 250,000 sweat glands and produce as much as a pint of moisture each day. An increase in body temperature will increase the perspiration level. Some people experience excessive perspiration of their feet. *Hyperhidrosis* is a medical term meaning excessive moisture. This moisture often increases the chance of blisters. Individuals with this condition may find that applying an antiperspirant to the feet reduces the amount of perspiration, which in turn prevents the formation of blisters. David Zuniga is one runner who has found that the use of an antiperspirant has helped his feet. He started using an antiperspirant on the recommendation of his podiatrist and finds his feet stay "dry as a bone."

Aside from antiperspirants, problems associated with excessive moisture can often be reduced by wearing moisture-wicking socks, changing socks frequently, and changing shoes if the moisture is particularly excessive.

To save your shoes from faster than normal deterioration from the excess moisture, sprinkle a bit of baking soda powder into each shoe after using them. Remove the insoles and shake the shoes to get the powder evenly distributed. The baking soda will also help control the harsh smells that are common with heavy sweating inside shoes.

Blisters & Antiperspirants

Ultrarunner Mike Palmer has worked at resolving blister problems related to sweaty feet. He wears sandals as much as he can to keep his feet dry during the day. A couple of weeks before an ultra of 50 miles or more, he uses alcohol at night to dry his feet. He has also found coating his feet with tincture of benzoin dries the skin and provides a protective coating. In the month before a 100-mile run, if the weather allows, he tries to frequently walk about a mile barefoot in an attempt to further toughen the skin. Then before the run he uses an absorbent foot powder and puts dispensers of this powder in his drop bags for every point where he will make a sock change. Mike also recommends frequent sock changes during long races. Even though this is time-consuming, it's better than trying to run on hot spots and blistered feet. For Mike, the moisture promotes blistering. Since using benzoin, the maceration (the whitish, flaky condition of moist skin) has been eliminated and blistering is not so frequent or extensive.

In an interesting study, cadets attending the U.S. Military Academy were separated into two groups that used either an antiperspirant or placebo preparation. Each group was asked to apply their preparation for five consecutive nights before completing a 21K hike. After the hike, only 21 percent of the cadets who reported using the antiperspirant preparation for at least three nights before the hike were diagnosed with foot blisters. The placebo group reported a 48 percent incidence of foot blisters. Joseph Knapik, ScD, the lead author of the study that appeared in the August 1998 issue of the *Journal of the American Academy of Dermatology* reported, "Blisters are usually minor problems, but they can cause great discomfort for the patient. Typically they only require simple first aid and a short period of limited activity. It is possible, however, for them to lead to more serious problems such as local or systemic infections."

Researchers theorized that reduced sweating might reduce friction and consequently lower the occurrence of blisters. The cadets applied the preparation to completely dry feet, up the ankle to the top of the boot line. Before the hike, each cadet was examined for existing foot conditions. Immediately after the hike, the feet of each cadet were inspected for blisters using the same criteria as the prehike examination. Researchers found that sweat reduction was a key mechanism for the reduction of blisters.

FOOT ANTIPERSPIRANT PRODUCTS

ANTIPERSPIRANTS that can work on your feet are available in drugstores. Check the shelves at your local store and try one or two. Rich Schick recommends using Drysol, a prescription-strength antiperspirant that is applied daily and after a couple days virtually eliminates all perspiration. Others have had success with Ban Roll-on.

BROMI-LOTION is a unique antiperspirant formulated as a soothing lotion, rather than as a spray or roll-on. It is available only by special order through your local drugstore, pharmacy, or podiatrist. **Gordon Laboratories, (800) 356-7870**

BROMI-TALC PLUS is an antiperspirant powder from Gordon Labs containing a deodorizing powder, sodium potassium, alumino silicate, bentonite, and talc to eliminate odor instantly and help reduce sweating of the feet. *See "Powder Products," page 91.*

DRYZ INSOLES help the feet stay dryer and cooler while eliminating odor. *See "Insole Products," page 60.*

FOOT SOLUTION, by Onox, is a spray solution made to control excessive moisture and foot odor. A combination of mineral salts decreases excessive sweat and foot odor symptoms. The spray also helps reduce blistering and itching while repelling athlete's foot fungus. Ingredients include zinc chloride, deionized water, sodium chloride, sodium nitrate, boric acid, and sodium silco-fluoride. Be aware that the salt solution will sting if you have cuts or breaks in your skin. Foot Solution can be ordered through Foot-Smart. **www.footsmart.com**

GOLD BOND is a medicated body powder. Use the extra-strength powder for maximum benefits in absorbing excessive moisture. *See "Powder Products," page 91.*

GORDON LAB'S NO. 5 FOOT POWDER is an antifungal aerosol spray that turns to powder once reaching the foot. It helps to decrease sweating, burning, and itching. *See Bromi-Talc in "Powder Products," page 91.*

ZEASORB is a super absorbent powder, absorbing six times it's weight in moisture and four time more than plain talcum powder. *See "Powder Products," page 91.*

While the antiperspirant was found to be very effective in reducing blisters, some side effects did occur. "Itching and rashes occurred in 57 percent of the antiperspirant group, but only 6 percent of the placebo group," Dr. Knapik noted. "This suggests that a large portion of the population may have problems with the antiperspirant used in the study. However, reducing the amount of the active compound or applying the antiperspirant every other night, rather than every night as the cadets did, may reduce the irritation."

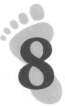

Taping for Blisters

I f your feet are prone to blistering, taping may be a lifesaver. After 12 hours of a 72-hour run, my Vaseline-coated feet were almost too sore to run on, and I had a blister between two toes. Nancy Crawford, an experienced running friend, taught me how to prepare my feet for taping and use duct tape to both fix the blister and tape the tender balls of my feet, which would likely blister in the hours ahead. I completed the next 60 hours without a foot problem!

While you may consider duct taping an extreme, consider the benefits of taping if you are highly susceptible to blisters. You can tape before your event as a proactive preventive measure or in a reactive mode after hot spots or blisters develop. Tape can be applied to more than feet. Rich Lewis finds that applying duct tape to his socks over where he typically develops hot spots or blisters, particularly in new shoes, is a good prevention measure. Others use duct tape inside their shoes or boots to cover irritating seams in their footwear.

Ultrarunner Gillian Robinson usually tapes her big toes because the skin underneath the toe almost always rubs. For a long ultra (100 miles) she tapes more extensively—all of her toes, the balls of her feet, and the arches. She typically does not have heel trouble. Don Lundell usually follows a specific regiment for short ultras: taping the places where he gets blisters (left foot: heel and inside of the foot behind the big toe). When he pretapes, he prefers the Denise Jones method (see below), using Elastikon and Micropore tapes.

Keep in mind that the overall goal of taping is prevention. While taping is a great skill to learn, you need to be sure the shoes you wear are the best fit possible for your feet. With shoes that fit well, your taping needs will hopefully be minimal.

I recommend that runners first train in the conditions for the race intended. Once a runner has trained in this environment, it becomes evident what areas of the feet are prone to problems and they can then be pre-taped. Just as training for the distance is vitally important, so is trying the technique of taping in training prior to the race.

Below are four methods of taping the feet. The first uses duct tape. The second method, devised by Suzi Cope, uses Johnson & Johnson Elastikon tape. The third, developed by Badwater Blister Queen Denise Jones, uses a combination of Elastikon and Micropore tapes. U.S. Army Captain Dave Hamilton learned the fourth method from Dutch Red Cross workers at the military's Nijmegen Four-Day March. Each method can be used with the other types of tape mentioned earlier. Following a description of each of these methods are descriptions of how to tape different parts of the feet. Remember, any tape that moves or shifts is worse than no tape at all.

Taping Basics

There are several types of tape available to try. Duct tape is the standard most often used, but Elastikon and Micropore have become popular with ultrarunners and adventure racers. HyTape, Kinesio Tex Tape, Leukotape, and Leukoplast can be used as well. (Athletic white tape is not well suited for taping feet.) The medical tapes can be found at or ordered through most medical supply stores or through Internet searches.

Types of Tape

DUCT TAPE is a 2-inch-wide, very sticky silver tape with a fabric core that has excellent adhesive qualities. It does not breathe but is very strong and tough. Buy high-quality duct tape, which is available at any hardware store.

ELASTIKON, from Johnson & Johnson Medical Inc., is a medium-thickness, stretchy, breathable tape that comes in 1-, 2-, 3-, and 4-inch widths.

HYTAPE is a pink tape with excellent adhesive properties. The ½-inch and 1-inch widths can be used for toes. It is nonporous.

KINESIO TEX TAPE is a ribbed tape that stretches bidirectionally. Designed for muscle taping, it comes in 2-, 3-, and 4-inch widths. This tape is breathable, and a water-resistant type is available.

LEUKOPLAST tape is a cloth, nonstretchy tape with an aggressive adhesive. The width used in the method described is ½ inch although it comes in other widths. It is sold in Europe but is hard to find in the U.S.

LEUKOTAPE P is a nonbreathable tape made by BSM Medical. It comes in one width, 1½ inch. It is strong and very sticky—a good choice as an alternative to duct tape.

MICROPORE is a paper tape made by 3M that comes in ½-inch and 1-inch widths. The tape needs to be applied over a tape adherent base in order to stick well.

Athletes who decide to try taping should purchase a tape adherent that provides a taping base to hold the tape to the skin (see "Skin Tougheners & Tape Adherents," page 96). The best adherents are Cramer Products' Tuf-Skin spray, Mueller's Tuffner Clear Spray, or tincture of benzoin in a liquid or swabs (a woman's blush makeup brush is a good size for applying the benzoin).

Preparation includes several steps. Before taping, clean the feet of their natural oils, dust, and dirt. This is vital to getting a good stick with the tape. If you have used any lubricant on your feet, wipe it off with a towel first. Rubbing alcohol works well to clean the feet and dries quickly. For fanny-pack use, buy alcohol wipes in small disposable packets. Next, apply the tape adherent to the areas needing taping and let it dry. Then apply the tape based on your specific needs or problems.

You can use a thin layer of a lubricant under the tape at problem areas like the ball of the foot or the heel. It will help with the removal of the tape. When it has been on awhile, it sometimes takes the skin off underneath it because that skin is soft. It hurts a lot if you peel that soft skin off with the tape. Duct tape is harder to get off and is more likely to take the skin with it, especially if it has been on a long while.

When applying the tape, keep it as smooth as possible. Ridges in the tape may cut into the skin and lead to irritation that may cause blisters. If the tape must be overlapped, be sure the overlapping edge of the tape is in the same direction as the force of motion. For example, if taping the ball of the foot, the force is towards the rear of the foot, so the most forward piece of tape should overlap over the piece towards the back. If taping the heel, the force is towards the rear and up the back of the heel, so the tape on the bottom of the heel should overlap the piece higher up on the back of the heel. This will keep the tape from catching on the sock and peeling up. The less overlap the better. Applying the tape too tightly may cause circulation problems. If, after application, the skin becomes discolored, cool, or numb, loosen the tape.

Place a single layer of toilet paper or tissue over any existing blisters where the outer skin has pulled loose from the inner skin. This keeps the adhesive from attacking the sensitive area and protects the blistered skin when the tape is removed. You can also substitute a piece of duct tape against the tissue, sticky side to sticky side, allowing the slick side of the duct tape to face the hot spot or blister. Try not to use gauze since it is too abrasive.

After the foot is taped, several finishing touches should be made. Run a thin layer of Bag Balm, Vaseline, or similar lubricant over the tape and around the edges. This reinforces the tape's status as part of your foot by providing a barrier that neutralizes any adhesive leaks and allows the taped surface to slip easily across friction points without snagging. Finally, after spraying and taping your feet, be sure to apply a sprinkling of powder to the sprayed areas that are not taped to counteract any adhesive left uncovered. Jane Moorhead saw a podiatrist using a votive candle and, after taping, rubbing it over the edges of the tape. The small amount of wax reduces friction and helps prevent curling. This is less messy than using Bag Balm or Vaseline.

You may be able to tape all areas of your feet yourself. If you have problems reaching the outer edges of your feet, your heels, or any other awkward area, find someone to help with the taping.

As important as taping the feet is, all those benefits can be lost if the athlete is not careful in putting on or taking off his or her socks. The socks should be rolled on and off. All the time and value of a good tape job can be ruined when changing socks too fast. The use of a shoehorn is recommended to keep addition fiction off the heel as it is lowered into the shoe.

When removing the tape, work slowly and carefully. You do not want to pull off a layer of skin or a toenail with the tape. Work from the sides to the center, using the fingers of one hand to hold the skin while pulling the tape with the other hand. Ultrarunner Suzi Cope suggests using baby oil and gentle massage to roll off the tape and excessive adhesive. You can use fingernail polish remover to get rid of any leftover adhesive on your skin or toenails. After a race, Will Brown gets in the shower with the tape still on. After it's wet, he lifts one side of the tape up so more water can get in. After a few minutes, it's easy to remove.

Taping is useful for prerun preparation as well as for fixing newly developed problem spots. If you typically blister on the balls of your feet, consider taping before the run when you have the time to do it right rather then at an aid station when you need every minute of time. Practice taping to learn how best to apply the tape to meet your particular needs. Determine how much time is needed to do a complete application. If you are going to have crew support for an event, teach them how to do the taping. It is usually easier to tape the night before an event than wait until the morning when time is rushed and you may do a hurried job.

If you are bothered by blisters and have found that powders and/or lubricants do not work, try the different tapes to find a tape and taping method that works for you. In the chapter on foot-care kits (page 312), you will find a list of taping materials to carry during your runs and hikes.

Duct Tape Techniques

Duct tape is tough. In 1968, *Popular Mechanics* reviewed Arno Adhesive's "duct tape" in their New Products column. They casually noted it was also ideal for "other jobs around the house." Little did they know that the silver duct tape would become a staple of the athlete's foot-care kit. A mail-order catalogue offers a T-shirt with a picture of the familiar silver roll and the words "When the Going Gets Tough, The Tough Use Duct Tape." Ultrarunner Ivy Franklin blistered so badly at the Arkansas Traveller 100 in 1994 that she dropped at 68 miles. Then she learned about the miracle of duct taping and ran the Umstead Trail 100 in 1995 and returned to the Arkansas Traveller 100 in 1996 without either blisters or hot spots.

Many runners have successfully used Gary Cantrell's article "From the South: The Amazing Miracle of Duct Tape"[16] to learn how to prevent and also to treat blisters. Gary's basic principle is to cover the spot that's injured with a patch, and in some cases then anchor the edges and corners of that patch. The powerful adhesive of duct tape holds it close and true to the outline of your skin and the tough plastic outer tape reinforced with fabric can withstand almost unlimited friction. The friction points on your skin will then have what amounts to an additional layer of skin—the duct tape. Gary's method follows, along with a few of my time-tested additions.

Remember a few general duct tape rules. Choose a good quality duct tape with a visible fabric core, not a cheap plastic imitation. Many hardware stores carry several different types of duct tape. The standard grade is typically 9-mil thick, while the contractor and professional grades are generally 10-mil. Duct tape is only available in a 2-inch width. Although the tape is sometimes available in a variety of colors, the common silver tape works the best.

Apply the tape over the danger spots where blisters frequently occur. Don't apply tape where it is not needed. Use only a single thickness since additional layers become too hard and unyielding. When the tape is applied, that part of the foot should be flexed to its maximum extension. Cut the ends of the tape so they are rounded. If your feet are hairy, shave the parts where the tape will be applied.

Generally speaking, with duct tape do not tape all the way around toes or the foot because of possible circulation problems. If after applying tape, the skin or portion of the foot farthest from the body becomes discolored, cool, or numb, loosen the tape.

Suzi Cope's Taping Techniques

Suzi Cope, an ultrarunner, developed this taping technique while completing the Grand Slam of trail ultrarunning, five 100-mile runs in one summer, with only a couple of small "tape" blisters. Suzi's technique involves taping the bottom of each foot up to the heel and around the sides of the foot and each toe. She recommends taping the night before an event, after taking a shower. She has often had the tape on up to 36 hours without a problem. River and stream crossings are not a problem since the tape is porous and dries as fast as socks and shoes. Suzi stresses this technique will not work for everybody. Your individual footprint and running style may affect the taping.

Suzi uses Johnson & Johnson's Elastikon tape in 2-inch and 4-inch widths. Do not stretch the tape, simply form it to the foot and press firmly. All points where the tape folds or is pinched together should be folded like gift wrap and cut flush with the skin. This is truly preventative maintenance, creating a sock type effect. Determine your specific hot spot or blister problems and try taping as needed. When cutting the tape flush with the skin, be careful not to cut the skin. She recommends baby oil and gentle massage to remove the tape.

Suzi technique uses the three steps to tape the whole foot. First she tapes the bottom of the foot, and then the sides, followed by the toes. If you only have problems on the ball of the foot, the heels, or the toes, use the appropriate taping strategy.

Denise Jones's Taping Techniques

Denise Jones's method uses Elastikon and Micropore tapes, with tincture of benzoin as an adherent. She also uses plenty of foot lubricant, usually Bag Balm and/or Hydropel.

To prepare feet for taping, Denise insists you have to file down any calluses with a pedicure file so that if a blister develops it can be treated. If thick calluses are allowed to remain, they can prove next to impossible to get underneath to drain blisters, and those blisters become larger and more painful. Before taping, also make sure toenails are trimmed square and filed so no rough edges remain.

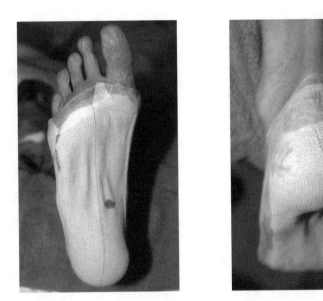

MATT FREDERICK

Effective use of Elastikon and Micropore tape.

Elastikon tape is stretchy, porous, and very sticky. It comes in the following widths: 1 inch (rarely used), 2 inch (used most often for balls of feet and heels), 3 inch (used for full bottom extending up and over heel about 1½ inches. Micropore comes in a 1-inch width that is occasionally used on the big toe. Otherwise, use the ½-inch width for the toes and also to seal the edges of Elastikon. Elastikon tape is not for toes—it's too abrasive. Recently Denise has tried Kinesio Tex Tape and likes its qualities. It can be

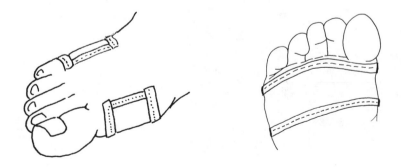

A typical use of two kinds of tape.

taped easily, it's very sticky, smooth, and stretchy, and it breathes. The only downside is that it's expensive. She has found that in extreme heat conditions, duct tape will not work and any tapes used need to be porous. Denise uses the following taping method:

> Most importantly, when I use Elastikon on the larger areas of the foot, it's imperative that tincture of benzoin is first swabbed onto the area where the edges will be. This sticks the edges of the tape to the foot. Allow the tincture to become tacky, and then tape as flatly and neatly as possible. Then, around the perimeter of the edges I use the ½-inch Micropore to seal the edges. Otherwise, I have found that the Elastikon tape rolls and creates a ridge that will blister. So, I stress that all Elastikon on the large areas of the foot are taped on the edges with Micropore tape. That means more tincture before placing the sealing of the edges. Micropore will not stick without tincture. Micropore tape is used on the toes, again preparing the toe with tincture first.

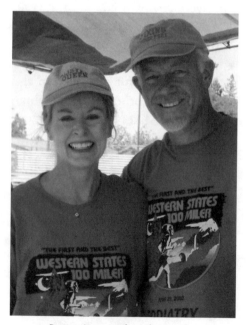

Denise Jones with author at the Western States 100-Mile Endurance Run.

If the ends of the toes blister, then I tape over the top of the toe first, then around the toe to encase it like a glove. I make sure that all areas of the toe are secure with no gaps and no ridges. If a corner is bulky, I cut it off and secure it with more tincture. If one toe is taped and the toe next to it is not, make sure the tape is absolutely smooth so that the rubbing that occurs in running will not blister the untaped toe. After taping, use foot powder to keep feet dry within the socks.

If taping over a blister, Denise first uses Zeasorb foot powder to dry the feet before taping, and then she cleans the feet with an alcohol wipe. After taping, she puts more powder over any exposed benzoin. You should use 2nd Skin over blisters, but cut a hole in each blister for draining. This allows the runner to continue with little pain. It's the fluid in the blister that causes the pain.

Denise recommends also using Silicone Glove by Avon underneath and before applying Elastikon on the large areas of the foot but not to the edges. This allows tape removal without tearing the edematous skin underneath.

Finally, pretape the night before a race and wear socks to bed to help the tape conform to the foot. If anything comes unstuck during the night, it can then be restuck.

Dutch Red Cross Taping Technique

The taping method learned by U.S. Army Captain Dave Hamilton, a physician's assistant, at the military Nijmegen Four-Day 140K March is actually used in that march as a post-injury treatment. The foot is cleaned and any blisters are treated. Then the skin is prepped with benzoin. The Dutch Red Cross workers used Leukoplast tape in ½-inch widths (this tape is hard to find in the U.S.). Dave emphasizes any other tape used should be cloth and nonstretchable. The method involves taping either the forefoot or the heel. Toes can be taped by one using methods covered later in this chapter.

To tape the forefoot, start at the base of the toes and apply the first piece of tape. Dave advises cutting the tape off the roll and applying it, and then cutting off any excess tape. Stick the tape to the center of the foot first, and then smooth it out towards the sides to ensure no wrinkles appear. Add another strip of tape, overlapping the previous strip by one-third. Continue to add strips until the foot is taped down to midfoot. Once the strips clear the toes, the end of each strip should stop on the top of the foot, just over the side of each foot. This creates a multilayered base of tape that is strong, tight, and protective. If there are any problems under the tape, the layers nearest the problem point can be peeled back to expose the blister and expel any fluid.

Tape the heel from the top of the Achilles tendon and work your way down to the midfoot. The tape is applied in the same manner as on the forefoot.

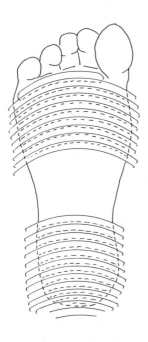

Dutch taping involves attaching overlapping strips of tape across the ball of the foot and heel.

After taping the feet, apply powder, and reapply powder when changing socks. It is important to carefully roll the socks on and off the foot to avoid pulling any of the tape loose.

The ½-inch width tape seems strange, but it allows easy replacement of any sections of tape and access to any blisters needing additional care. The importance of the nonstretch tape is to provide support to the natural contours of the foot and provide a slick surface when coated with powder.

If blisters are present, Dave treats them using DuoDerm, a wound dressing and then tapes over the DuoDerm. This blister patching method is detailed in the chapter on treating blisters in the section on advanced blister care (page 214).

Taping the Feet

A good tape job is an art. It takes practice. Denise Jones warns,

If taping isn't done properly, it's almost worse than no taping. Any rough edge can become a subsequent blister. Some of the [athletes] I've worked on have used Elastikon, but [they] either didn't seal the edges with Micropore or didn't even use a tape adherent at all. Then the tape rolled. I've tried so hard to get the message out there, but when I see the job of taping that is done, it's less than adequate, and sometimes even a setup for blistering, for example, too close to the toe junction on the balls of the feet, so blisters develop between the toes once the feet swell.

So practice early, and practice often. Develop taping skills with each part of your foot. And then practice on your friends and with your teammates.

Ball of the Foot

The easiest method of taping the ball of the foot is to take a long strip of full-width tape and place it, adhesive side up, on the floor. Place your foot on it at a right angle, with the trouble spot dead center on the tape. Then flatten your foot to make it as wide as possible and pull the ends of the tape up, either overlapping them on the top of your foot or cutting them an inch up on either side of the foot. Cut the tape at the forward edge of the ball of the foot so it does not contact or cut into the crease at the base of the toes or the toes themselves.

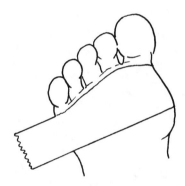

Cut tape to conform to the shape of the foot. Then lay tape sticky side up on the floor and step onto it with your full weight.

Some athletes may find it easier to make a card template the shape of their foot—from the ball of the foot to the base of the toes. Then cut the tape according to the template. This makes trimming easier, if needed at all, especially if you are taping your own feet.

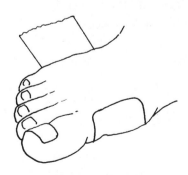

Wrap tape up the sides of the foot.

Bottom of the Foot

Suzi and Denise both advocate taping the bottom of the foot from the ball of the foot to the heel. Apply a 4-inch piece of Elastikon tape from just behind the bend of the toe base, centering the tape on the bottom of the foot from front to back. Have equal edges on the inside and outside of the foot. Trim the front edge to follow the contour of the toe base, avoiding the crease. Bring the back edge up the heel and fold over on each side, like a gift wrap, making a dart. Cut the fold flush with the foot, leaving two edges just meeting in a V pattern. Next, tape the side of the feet.

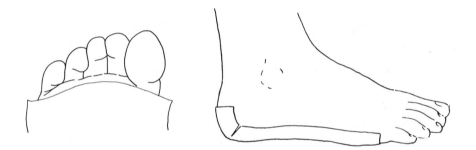

Center the foot across the width of the tape, allowing equal amounts to wrap up both sides. Cut the front edge to conform to the curve of the forefoot, and mold up the heel, cutting off extraneous tape creases.

Sides of the Foot

Once the 4-inch piece of tape is affixed to the bottom of the foot, Suzi then adds tape to the sides of the foot. Apply a 2-inch piece around the foot from one side to the other. Slightly overlap the edge of the 4-inch tape. Trim the edges to avoid rubbing at the toe crease and anklebone.

Apply a single strip of tape around the back of the heel, overlapping the edges of the piece attached to the foot bottom.

If you find the bottom edge of the tape catching on your socks, put this layer on before taping the bottom of the foot. Then tape the bottom of the foot so that tape overlaps the side of the foot tape. This method keeps the overlapping tape in the direction of the force of motion as described earlier.

Bottom of the Heel

Remember when applying tape to the bottoms of your feet or heels to grasp the toes of the foot and pull back to stretch the skin to its fullest. Otherwise as you run or walk, the shear forces will loosen the tape and may cause additional blisters.

Start with a large patch of tape covering the entire heel; attach it with both the foot and ankle flexed forward and up (pull your toes toward your shin). Take a long strip of 1-inch width tape (or cut to a 1-inch width), cover the forward edge of the patch under your foot, and bring the ends up to overlap on top of the foot. Take another medium strip, cover the edge on the back of your heel, and bring the ends around the ankle to overlap on top of the first strip. When applying the tape, lay the strips on the skin. Applying them too tightly can impair circulation.

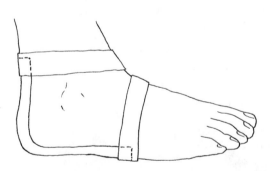

Attach tape from the middle of the foot bottom and up the back of the heel. Secure it with one strip of tape encircling the arch and another around the ankle.

Sides of the Heel

Many times, feet blister at the area where the insole meets the inside of the shoe. The side of the heel can be taped by either running a piece of tape around the back of the heel or under the heel from side to side. With either method, cut the tape into a V as necessary to avoid folds in the tape. Try to avoid taping over the two anklebones.

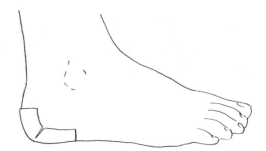

Taping problem areas that often occur along the sides of the heel.

The Toes

Gillian Robinson suggests if you tape any toes, it will probably work better to tape them all and avoid the rubbing of taped toes against untaped ones. Be careful not to tape too tightly since that can cause other problems. Also, don't tape too close to where your toes meet your feet.

Suzi Cope tapes toes with pieces of the 2-inch Elastikon tape. Denise Jones recommends ½ inch or 1 inch Micropore, because she finds the Elastikon is too abrasive to the other toes. The Micropore paper tape is so thin that it goes on easy, is simple to patch if necessary, and actually holds up well.

Tape only the last two joints, avoiding the crease at the base of the toes. Roll the tape around the toe, overlapping over the toenails for a double-layer but keeping a single-layer on the sides of the toes. Fold the excess over at the tips of the toes, pinching the top and bottom together. Since Elastikon tape is stretchy, the overlapping of the tape is not an issue here as it is with duct tape. Cut off any wrinkles or corners of the tape with sharp scissors, so it conforms to your toe perfectly. After the entire toe is covered like a glove, apply with the swab another layer of the tincture to seal the tape ends. When the toes are finished, bend them back and forth to make sure they feel good and not restricted.

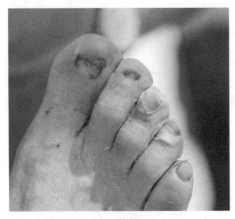

Toe blisters can be challenging to patch.

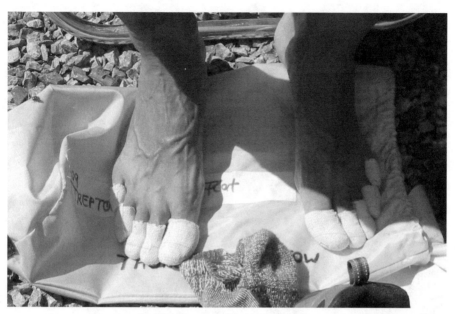

Ten Elastikon-taped toes, ready to go.

A proper taping on toes or larger areas should appear like an extra layer of skin on the foot—no lumps or bumps. If any corners bunch anywhere, pinch them together and cut excess flush with small scissors. Sometimes tincture needs to be applied again to keep corners and edges down.

The alternative method of taping toes is a two-piece tape job. First, tear off a small strip and use it to wrap from the base of the toenail around the tip of the toe and to the bottom of the toe even with the end on top, leaving two free ends. (Omit this step for toes that don't blister at the tip.) Wrap another strip around the circumference of the toe, covering the free ends of the first strip, if it was used. Have the two ends meet but be sure to try to

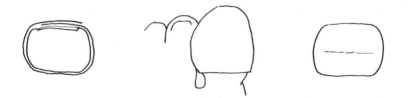

Use one piece of tape to encircle the toe, pinch it closed, and cut it flush with the skin.

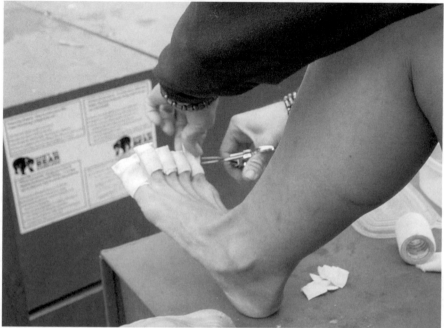

Catra Corbett-McNeely taping her toes.

avoid overlapping them on top of the toe. Always use a large enough strip to cover the toe's "knuckle joint" so that both outside edges are too small to slide over the joint and cause the tape to bunch off or slip off the end of the toe. Never extend the edge far enough down that it will dig into the tender skin between the toes. For taping against toenail friction, tape the receiving toe, rather than the offending nail.

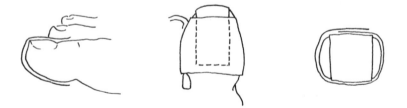

An alternative method is to use two pieces of tape, the first attached from the top of the toe over the tip to the bottom, and the second encircling the toe.

Between the Toe & Foot

This important method comes in handy for those hard-to-tape areas at the base of your toes or between the toes. Cut a small blister pad of your choice and place it firmly over the area or blister. Fasten it in place with a slightly larger square of tape. Take a long thin strip of tape and run it diagonally, corner to corner, between your toes from the top of your foot to the ball of your foot. Take another long, thin strip and do the

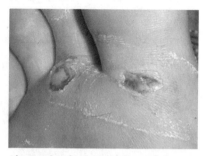

Blisters that form at the base of the toes can be the hardest to tape effectively.

same with the two remaining corners. Now you have a pad on the blister, the pad protected by tape, and the whole thing held firmly in place by the four strips attaching the corners to the tops and bottoms of your feet. Now, anchor these strips with the single piece described for the ball of the foot, and the most difficult blister of all is fixed.

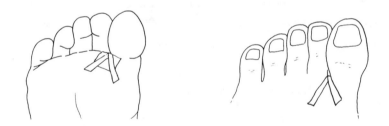

Two diagonal strips of tape anchor the patch over a blister.

TAPING ALTERNATIVE PRODUCTS

BUNGA Toe Pads and Toe Caps are made from a medical-grade polymer material. **Absolute Athletics, (888) 286-4272, www.bungapads.com**

BUNHEAD GEL products are made of a nonsilicone polymer, formulated with medical grade mineral oils to cushion and protect those areas of the foot prone to friction trauma. They are washable, supple, comforting, hypoallergenic, and nontoxic. Styles include Jelly Tips, Jelly Toes, the Big Tip, and a really Big Tip designed for big toes. Locate a retailer through their Website. **www.bunheads.com**

ENGO PERFORMANCE PATCHES are made of a thin fabric-film composite that can greatly reduce friction in targeted locations within your footwear. The patches give a slick, slippery surface to the area of your footwear or insole where friction is a problem. The adhesive creates a strong bond, eliminating migration, even through moisture and sweat. When used for hotspots, blister formation is prevented. If used to help treat a blister, healing time is significantly decreased. Patches come in three sizes: small ovals, large ovals, and sheets, and they can be trimmed for a custom fit. Each patch is *extremely* durable, lasting anywhere from several weeks to several months. **Tamarack Habilitation Technologies Inc., (763) 795-0057, www.goengo.com**

HAPAD offers PediFix Visco-Gel Toe Caps that can be used over toes to prevent blisters. **Hapad, (800) 544-2723, www.hapad.com**

PRO-TEC'S TOE CAPS, made from custom-grade silicone, are soft and stretchable to fit all toes. Locate a reseller through their Website. **www.pro-tecathletics.com**

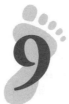

Orthotics

Orthotics are custom-made or over-the-counter insoles that replace the generic, removable insoles in store-bought shoes and boots. Their purpose is to cure athletes' lower extremity ailments. Many runners wear an orthotic device in one or both shoes to help maintain the foot in a functionally correct position. Orthotics may be prescribed for the treatment of plantar fasciitis, tendinitis, knee pain, shin splints, lower-back pain, Morton's neuromas, and other conditions. Orthotics can correct gait irregularities and provide support for flat feet and pronation problems. They can also relieve pressure by providing support behind a problem area such as a callous, neuroma, or metatarsal injury. Mal-alignment problems such as leg-length inequality can also be corrected. Typically prescribed by a podiatrist or orthopedist, orthotics are medical devices made from cast impressions of your feet. A properly fit orthotic will control arch and pressure-point problems.

Signs that you may need an orthotic can include repeated overuse strains or injuries, excessive fatigue in your legs and feet, genetic structural problems (over- or under-pronation, bunions, differences in leg length, arch problems, etc.), or your shoes show different wear patterns or wear out quicker than usual. The need for orthotics may begin with pain in your feet, repeated blistering in the same place on your feet from pressure, or even problems in your knees or hips as your gait is changed due to biomechanical stresses. Doug Mitchell says he "had substantial pain in the ball/metatarsal area many years ago. I was doing about 60 miles a week and heavy lifting, too, including very heavy calf raises. It turned out I had a minor structural problem in the foot that created a lot of stress on the ball of my feet. After a while, I went to see a podiatrist, which resulted in my first orthotics. They solved the problem." Doug uses his orthotics almost exclusively in his running and athletic footwear. Check with your health-care plan to determine if they cover orthotics.

An added benefit of orthotics is the way they support the body's natural movements. This reduces the demands placed on the muscles when the body is out of alignment. The result is less work by the muscles, which translates to less fatigue, fewer injuries, and higher performance.

When you work with your pedorthist, podiatrist, or orthopedist to determine the right orthotic for your feet, remember several key points:

- Talk to your podiatrist about soft, semirigid, and rigid designs.
- Fiber-reinforced orthotics are typically stronger than other types.
- Make sure your shoes will accommodate the orthotics. This may depend on the depth of the uppers and the design of the inside of the shoe.
- Determine whether your orthotics are to be used alone or with your shoe's stock insole.
- If possible, have a padded layer of material added to the top of the orthotic or use a flat Spenco insole on top of the orthotics in your shoe for cushioning.
- If you change the model of shoes you wear, have the orthotics adjusted to fit the new shoes.
- Ascertain whether the orthotics are for short- or long-term use. This will depend on your reason for needing them.

Typical Orthotic Modifications & Alterations

- Extra-deep heel seat for more rear-foot control
- Extra heel cushioning
- Soft forefoot extensions at the end of toes

- Metatarsal pads, either soft or pressed into the shell, which can take pressure off neuromas and metatarsal pain
- Morton's extension for a short first metatarsal/long second
- Extra varus (roll out)/valgus (roll in) forefoot or rear foot posting, which inverts or everts the foot more
- Cutouts in the extension for relieving pressure

Custom-Made Orthotics

Custom-made orthotics may be soft, semirigid, or rigid, and are made specifically for your feet. Materials may include felt pads, cork, foam, viscoelastic, silicon, closed-cell rubber or closed-cell polyethylene, fiberglass, carbon fiber, or leather. Orthotics can be made in various lengths and include metatarsal pads or heel wedges. They are made to work in partnership with your boots and shoes. Poor-quality boots and shoes may alter the corrective action of an orthotic.

In the article "The Ideal Running Orthosis: A Philosophy of Design,"[17] the authors build a case for the ideal orthotic. They recommend a custom fit in either semirigid or semiflexible design, lightweight, yet inexpensive, with a covering to decrease shear while giving control to both the forefoot and hind foot, all while retaining memory in its shape and being adjustable at a later time. It also needs to be transferable to most of the client's shoes. They place orthotics in two categories of design: corrective and accommodative. A *corrective* orthotic should attempt, with a rigid design, to correct the foot's position so that its abnormal anatomy will mold to the corrected position. An *accommodative* orthotic should attempt to relieve areas of high stress or reposition the foot to better deal with its stress, usually with a soft or semiflexible design. The most common type of orthotic is semiflexible.

Getting Orthotics

Orthotics can be made, ordered, and casted by many professionals: physical therapists, trainers, physician's assistants, pedorthists, orthopedic techs, chiropractors, and podiatrists, to name a few. Given a choice, I would recommend that a sports podiatrist be the ordering and casting professional, with a pedorthist as the second choice. Finding the professional who has the patience to listen to your history is important. There are some other professionals that do a fine job diagnosing and casting for orthotics, but feet are a podiatrist's primary interest unlike the others listed above.

Whoever makes your orthotics needs to ask the right questions and order the right tests to make the correct diagnosis about which type of

All Orthotics Are Not Alike

Custom-molded orthotics are devices made from an actual mold or cast of the foot. There are two mediums to cast in, foam and plaster splints. Foam is neater, but is inaccurate. Impressions are usually taken with the patient seated. Once the material is compressed, it cannot be changed. Too much pressure in one area and the casting is flawed. Plaster splints allow for the foot to be manipulated into the correct position while the material is still soft. The cast then hardens over the next two to four minutes. Impressions are either taken with the patient sitting with the legs straight out to the caster or lying prone (stomach down) with feet dangling off the end of a table. This author prefers the later.

The majority of orthotics that are used for sports are made from white polypropylene or any one of the many varieties of carbon fiber. Carbon-fiber orthotics may be flexible or ultra rigid. If adjustments such as raising or lowering the arch or removing a high spot are needed, the carbon-fiber varieties are easily adjusted by heating with a heat gun and then manipulating. They hold their adjustment much better than the polypropylenes that have a lot more memory. These devices tend to go back to their original shape after attempted heat adjustments. Permanent adjustments have to be made by the maker of the orthotic.

The stiffness of the orthotic is an important feature. The more flexible devices provide less control but can be more comfortable. These are ideal when an accommodative forefoot or metatarsal pad is used. Though if control is what is needed to prevent excess movement such as over-pronation or over-supination, then a rigid device will normally be well tolerated. I can't even begin to count the number of times I have replaced another doctor's flexible orthotics with a pair of semirigid or rigid ones with great success.

— Podiatrist Tim Jantz

corrective orthotic is necessary. The typical process includes a detailed injury history, complete lower-extremity biomechanical examination including a gait analysis, and a check of your shoes or boots. The aim is to identify the cause of your injury and try to prevent its continuation or recurrence. *Patient compliance in wearing the orthotic is the dominant issue in resolving foot problems.* Modifications to the orthotics may be necessary to ensure a proper fit—if the orthotic is uncomfortable, chances are you won't wear it. Once you are using orthotics without any pain, continue to use the orthotics as long as they work for your feet. Some injuries that require orthotics will be relieved after a short period of time; other gait, support, and foot-function problems will require long-term use.

Ask your pedorthist, podiatrist, or orthopedist what you need to do to help the orthotics work. You should receive complete instructions on the use and care of your orthotics. He or she may give you a detailed treatment schedule of stretching and strengthening exercises and advice on shoe or boot selection. You may also be advised to wear the orthotics for several hours a day and gradually work your way up to longer periods.

If your foot seems to slip on your orthotic, ask about changing the surface material. A thin layer of Spenco insole material or your favorite insole material can usually be glued to the orthotic using rubber cement. The use of Spenco's Slip-In Insoles can add needed cushioning to your orthotics. Check with the maker of your orthotic before adding anything to the surface since doing so may change your gait and affect the purpose of the orthotic.

If you have orthotics that are three-quarter length, basically stopping at the ball of the foot, you need to use a thin insole, similar to the green Spenco flat insoles, under the orthotic. Usually running or hiking on the exposed bottom of the shoe is uncomfortable. Ask the maker of your orthotic how to add cushion under the forefoot and toes.

Mail-order orthotics need to be checked out thoroughly and purchased only through reputable companies. Adjustments to mail-order orthotics can be difficult. Arch supports sold in sporting goods and drugstores should not be mistaken for orthotics. The Hapad, Lynco, and Spenco orthotics identified below are just three of many low-cost orthotics that can be helpful as an alternative to custom orthotics and "quick-fix" drugstore remedies.

Over-the-Counter Orthotics

Not everyone needs a custom orthotic, and it may be worth your while to try one or two over-the-counter insoles. They may work. Some of these insoles are designed for specific foot problems. Ultrarunner and podiatrist Tim Jantz explains:

> Store-bought orthotics are just that—they are purchased at a store such as Wal-Mart, Kmart, Osco, Walgreens, or running specialty stores. These devices I refer to as 'arch supports.' They support the arch, which can provide relief of mild arch strain and heel pain to name a few. But they don't address the biomechanical problems that often are the cause of many maladies. They are simple, soft, and flexible. After all, they are made to fit every foot type that is a size 8 or 10 or 12. Some examples are Sof-Sole and Dr. Scholl's Dyna Step. These types of devices consist of soft to firm foam, and some even have a thin layer of carbon fiber for more support. They range in price from $5 to $35.

Nick Williams tells how he "had tried hard orthotics, soft orthotics, Spenco orthotics, and just about anything else to keep my feet from hurting." Then an orthopedic surgeon told him about Hapads and gave him a pair. They have kept him pain free for the last five years and are flexible on trails. Nick now swears by Hapads and via email told ultrarunner Ed Furtaw about them. Ed wore custom-made orthotics for 10 years but now uses the Comf-Orthotic three-quarter–length insoles without heel pain. He says, "They are definitely more comfortable than wearing orthotics." Ed added Hapad Scaphoid Pads for extra arch support. Now Ed's wife has switched from custom orthotics to the Comf-Orthotic. After an area on one arch got a little sore, they peeled away some of the wool material to make it fit better. Ed believes that "with something like Hapads, a person can take more responsibility for their own orthotic adjustments, which would be very difficult or impossible with custom-molded rigid orthotics." An orthopedist told me that if he had only one product to offer his patients, he would choose Hapads!

ORTHOTIC PRODUCTS

Many custom-made orthotics are available, and your pedorthist, podiatrist, or orthopedist will help select the correct one for your feet. The product lines of custom-made orthotics and insoles are constantly changing.

ARCHCRAFTERS CUSTOMCOMFORT INSOLES are computer machined to the exact shape of your foot. Placing your feet into a specially designed "foot-printer" captures the imprint of your feet. A scanned image of your feet is then made from the imprint and is used to make your custom insoles. **ARCH Crafters, (877) 356-0010, www.archcrafters.com**

The insoles listed below are proven alternatives to the more costly custom orthotics. Your podiatrist or pedorthist can show you other types.

APEX FULL-LENGTH ANTI-SHOX SPORTS ORTHOTICS are molded with patented heel cushion, medial posting, longitudinal arch support, and metatarsal relief. Gel protects calcaneus and metatarsal heads. An antishear top cover holds the foot in place. **APEX Foot Health Industries, (800) 526-APEX, www.apexfoot.com**

The **EZ RUNNER ORTHOTIC** is a lightweight, thin-profile, fluid orthotic. Silicone fluid is sealed into a polyurethane pouch with a viscosity matching that of the foot's fat pad. Gel flows precisely with each stride from heel strike to push off. It provides cushioning and correction at the forefoot and metatarsal heads. **Performance Clinic, (866) 371-8897, www.footpainfree.com**

HAPAD ORTHOTICS are either full-length or three-quarter-length insoles. Both are made from Hapad featherweight wool. The coiled, springlike wool fibers provide firm and resilient support while offering arch, metatarsal, and heel cushioning. The full-length contoured Comf-Orthotic Sports Replacement Insole is made in three layers: a moisture-wicking suede top, a ventilated Poron middle layer for shock absorption, and a bottom of Microcel "Puff," a self-molding footbed. The insole includes a metatarsal bar to relieve pressure at the ball of the foot, a medial arch support to limit pronation, and a heel cup for stability and control of the foot and ankle. **Hapad, Inc., (800) 544-2723, www.hapad.com**

ORTHOTIC PRODUCTS

LYNCO BIOMECHANICAL SPORTS ORTHOTICS, made by Apex, offer a "ready-made" triple-density orthotic system that comes in enough variations to accommodate 90 percent of foot disorders. After identifying your foot type as normal, high arched, or flat/over-pronated, they create a model. Each model comes with either a neutral-cupped heel or a medial posted heel, and with or without a metatarsal pad. Additional Reflex self-adhesive pads can be added to the orthotics to relieve pain from Morton's toe, sesamoiditis, and leg-length discrepancy. **APEX Foot Health Industries, (800) 526-APEX, www.apexfoot.com**

PERFORMANCE SHOE SYSTEMS specializes in custom-molded orthotics and shoe conversions. The orthotics are made from a mold of your feet and can be used in any shoe. The shoe conversion turns your comfortable running shoes into professional cleats, which provide better support and comfort than off-the-shelf cleats. **Performance Shoe Systems, (909) 886-3842, www.performanceshoesystems.com**

POWERSTEPS INSOLES, by Dr. Les Appel, offer a unique four-phase design to relieve heel and arch pain. With a heel cradle and platform, a strong pre-scription-like arch support, an antibacterial top fabric, and a double layer cushion casing, they provide optimal arch and heel support and stability. **Stable Step, (888) 237-3668, www.powersteps.com**

SOLE CUSTOM FOOTBEDS, which use "heat to fit" technology, offer an excellent, inexpensive alternative to custom orthotics. They come in regular and ultra-cushioning versions. The footbeds have Poron cushioning, a deep heel cup for stability, and an aggressive arch for support. When you heat the insoles in your oven, put them into your shoes, and stand on them, they mold to your feet. **Edge Marketing Sales, (866) 235-7653, www.yoursole.com**

SPENCO ARCH SUPPORTS are offered in several designs. Their Orthotic Arch Support is heated in hot water and then shaped to your foot. Other designs are readymade for your foot size. **Spenco Medical Corporation, (800) 877-3626, www.spenco.com**

10

Gaiters

usually tell athletes of their foot-care options and advise them to make the best choice—however, I have two absolutes. The first: You should always use moisture-wicking socks. The second: If you are going out on trails, you need to wear gaiters.

A few years ago I was working an aid station at a 50K trail run, and I was amazed at how few runners wore gaiters. One thing was certain—all had muddy shoes and many had muddy socks. And I don't mean a few drops of mud. I mean the gooey, down your shoes and between your toes type of mud. The mud hardens, causes friction and hot spots, and blisters form. The pace slows, good running form dissolves, your biomechanics alter your stride, and the downhill spiral begins.

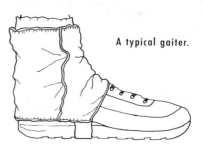

A typical gaiter.

Gaiters have been proven to be functional trail gear that all dedicated trail runners and adventure racers should use on trails. Hikers wearing low-top boots could also benefit from using gaiters. Forming a barrier around the leg and the top of the shoe, gaiters keep rocks, dust, and water-borne grit from getting into socks or between the socks and shoe. Gaiters can mean the difference between finishing a trail run or long hike with feet in good shape or feet plagued with hot spots and blisters. Most gaiters close on the side or in the front with Velcro.

My infatuation with gaiters began in 1989. Before my third Western States 100-Mile Endurance Run, I knew I had to do something extra to help my feet. Since I was prone to blisters and the trail was known for its dust and rocks, I decided to make a pair of gaiters. My homemade

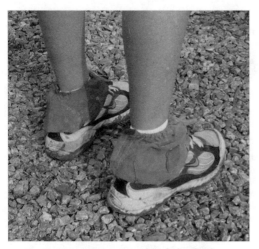

Gaiters are now considered standard gear for trail runners.

gaiters are described below. While I realize the gaiters alone did not make the whole difference, I did lower my personal best time by 1½ hours. The bottom line was that my feet were protected from the dust, grit, and rocks of the trail, and I had minimal problems.

Whether you are an adventure racer, a simple short-distance trail runner, a hiker, or an ultrarunner, you owe it to yourself to cover your socks and shoes with gaiters.

Making Your Own Gaiters

You can find any number of gaiters at your local stores. But sometimes, homemade ones work just all well or even better. Homemade gaiters can be easily made for running shoes or boots out of a pair of regular white crew socks. Pull the socks on your feet and with a scissors, cut the socks around the foot at the top of the shoe line. Toss out the foot portions. Fold the top of the sock down on itself so the folded down top covers the top of the shoe. Make a small hole in this folded down top at the back of the shoe and just to the rear of each upper shoe lace eyelet. Use an ice pick or the point of a scissors to make a small hole for the twist tie. Through the shoe hole place a plastic twist tie from a loaf of bread or similar package. By twisting the ties through these matching holes you have effectively covered the top of the shoes. Undo the twist ties to change shoes or socks while leaving the sock gaiter on your leg.

Ultrarunner Raymond Zirblis wore women's knee-highs over his shoes during the Marathon des Sables. The nylons stretched well, covered the whole shoe and up the leg, and kept sand and pebbles out, but the mesh was too open to keep dust out. They tore and wore away, but they stayed on all day. Ray used a fresh pair each day, reporting that while not perfect, they worked better than most of the gaiters he saw there during the six days of the desert run. Cathy Tibbetts-Witkes has also run the Marathon des Sables, and after much experimenting, she too designed her own gaiters. Custom-made from nylon, they attach to the soles of her shoes. After trying different designs and methods, she has sand proof gaiters.

Custom-Made Gaiters

Cathy Tibbetts-Witkes's gaiters are handmade by Cathy in two sizes, ankle-length for the ordinary ultra and knee-length for sand dunes in races such as the Marathon des Sables. They fit snugly over the shoe and attach to the outside with Velcro glued near the bottom on the sole of the shoe. Tibbetts-Witkes likes to make her own with 70 to 80 denier uncoated nylon, but other materials work as long as they are breathable. Her gaiters are held up with elastic sewn into the top that is sized for the circumference of the leg either above the ankle or calf. "It took a few tries to work the bugs out," Tibbetts-Witkes says, "but now I have totally sand-proof gaiters. Just keeping the fine dust out has cut down tremendously on blisters." Anyone interested in ordering a custom pair can contact her at cdtibbetts@yahoo .com. You'll have to show up at her home in New Mexico, but if you're in the neighborhood she'll schedule you for a fitting.

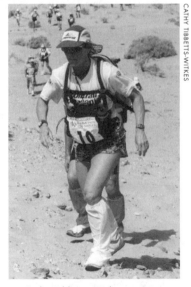

CATHY TIBBETTS-WITKES

Cathy Tibbetts-Witkes wearing her custom-made gaiters in the Marathon des Sables.

Kent Holder tells of using the arms off an old nylon jacket with elastic sleeves. He cuts the sleeves off about 6 inches up the sleeve from the cuff. He simply pulls the arms, elastic end first, onto his legs over his socks. The loose nylon covers the top of the shoes, and Kent reports it keeps 100 percent of the usual trail debris from entering the shoe. With this type of gaiter, there are no straps, so changing your shoes and socks is a breeze. He suggests looking for old nylon jackets at your local thrift store.

Rodney Hammons has found another way to get a gaiter effect. He wears a pair of knee-high type nylons under his Ultimax socks and then pulls the nylons down over the socks and tops of his shoes. Improvising can work wonders.

Repairing Gaiter Straps

The nylon straps or cords that come with most gaiters go under the shoes and boots and will wear out over time as the trails and rocks take their toll. Wrapping the straps with duct tape can help extend their life span. Then simply replace the tape when it wears through.

TIP: A Simple Slit Saves the Strap

Some athletes use a serrated-edge file or a knife to make a slit in the sole into which the strap or cord fits. This can protect them from fraying or being worn through as quickly. If you choose to make this modification to your shoes, be careful not to cut too deeply and compromise the integrity of the sole.

There are several methods for replacing the worn-out straps.

The nylon straps or cords that come with most gaiters go under the shoes and boots and will wear out over time as the trails and rocks take their toll. Wrapping the straps with duct tape can help extend their life span. Then simply replace the tape when it wears through. There are several methods to replace the worn out straps.

The first method simply uses ¼-inch nylon cord. Cut the old strap ¾-inch from its attachments to the gaiter. Use a lighted match to slightly melt the ends of the straps to prevent fraying. Be careful to not touch the melted nylon until it cools. Punch a small hole in the middle of the ¾-inch section, and use another lighted match to slightly melt the edges of the hole. Thread the nylon cord through the holes and knot securely so the length is the same as the old strap. Slightly melt the ends of the cord to avoid fraying.

Another method recommended by Mike Erickson uses swagged (pressed around the edges of the cable) ¹⁄₁₆-inch stainless steel cable instead of the nylon cord—he reports these have held up for over five years. Put a piece of duct tape over the swagged ends. Mike also reports using thin nylon cord doused with super glue and then wrapped with a couple layers of duct tape. Others use Kevlar shoelaces or picture-frame wire. Improvise to find other creative methods.

Do-it-Yourself Strap Replacement

To replace the nylon strap itself, use the method recommended by ultrarunner Kirk Boisseree, using the following materials, which are usually found in fabric stores: 1-inch-wide nylon webbing, size 24 (⅝-inch) metal large snaps (four sets of male and female pieces), and a snap installation tool. The snap tool can usually be found in craft or sewing stores. Make the new straps as follows:

1. Using the old strap as a guide, cut two pieces of webbing the same length.

2. Use a lighted match to slightly melt the ends of the straps to prevent fraying. Be careful to not touch the melted nylon until it cools.

3. At each end of the replacement straps, install a female snap.

4. Use a center punch or a nail to make a hole in the center of the strap ¾ inch from each end.

5. Push the snap through the hole and set the snap using the tool, following the instructions on the package.

6. Repeat for all four female snaps, making sure the snaps face the same way on each strap end.

7. Install the male snaps on the old straps about ½ inch to ¾ inch from the gaiter.

8. Using the center punch and installation tool, center the male snap in the hole, facing the outside of the shoe and set the snap.

9. Remove the middle portion of the worn strap, cutting it down to about a ½ inch from the new snaps.

10. Snap on the new straps and check for a proper fit.

GAITER PRODUCTS

JOETRAILMAN GAITERS are made without the usual strap under the shoe. They attach to the shoelaces closest to the front of the shoe via a hook and to the rear with a Velcro tab. The tension of the four-way stretch material holds the gaiter in place. Joe Dana's gaiters are offered in small and regular to fit all types of shoes. This style slips on your foot before putting on your shoes, which also makes it easy to changes shoes or socks. **http://home.att.net/~joe trailman/index.html**

NORTH FACE GAITERS come in two designs. The Scree Gaiters are made with a two-way stretch mono mesh. The Winter Gaiters GTX are made with stretch Gore-Tex that provides waterproof and breathable protection. Both form-fitting, pull-on styles come with hook attachment and a single-handed-drawstring closure system. Although their gaiters are made to fit several North Face shoes, they can be adapted to other shoes. **The North Face, www.thenorthface.com**

GAITER PRODUCTS

OUTDOOR RESEARCH makes several gaiter styles appropriate for running and hiking. Terra Gaiters are a light and tight scree gaiter made with woven SolarLite fabric designed to keep out dirt, dust, burrs, and muck when you're moving fast. The one-size-fits-all Flex-Tex Low Gaiters are made from stretchy Spandura fabric, suited for hiking boots or running shoes. One-size-fits-all Rocky Mountain Low Gaiters are made from vapor-permeable uncoated pack cloth, and the full-length Rocky Mountain High Gaiters are available in either Gore-Tex fabric or pack cloth. All gaiters open in the front with Velcro, have an eyelet on either side for a lace that goes under the shoe's arch, and a metal hook that fastens to a shoelace. **Outdoor Research, (888) 4OR-GEAR, www.orgear.com**

RACEREADY TRAIL GAITERS are made for running shoes and low-top hiking boots. Made in a combination of colors from quick-drying and breathable Supplex nylon, these gaiters have a "space-age tough" cord that goes under the shoe's arch. They fasten with the usual Velcro closure on the outside of the shoe. They could be used on other hiking boots by lengthening the strap. **RaceReady, (800) 537-6868, www.raceready.com**

REI makes several designs of gaiters. Their Desert Gaiters are made from Solarweave fabric for coolness. The Spring Gaiters are made with abrasion resistant Schoeller Dynamic Extreme fabric, and the Trail Gaiters are made with Cordura nylon. Each style has side Velcro closure and an instep cord. **Local REI stores or at www.rei.com**

VJ GAITERS are over-the-calf gaiters perfect for orienteering and cross-country trekking. A full-length zipper up the back makes them easy to use. A pad protects the shin. Made with Spandex nylon, they attach to the shoe laces at the front of the shoe and have a drawstring to secure them over the calf. **Orienteering Supplies, (866) 424-8377, www.866gaiters.com**

WESTERN STATES 100 TRAIL GAITERS are for running shoes. They are made of nylon Cordura fabric with a light urethane coating. A snap on each side of the gaiter attaches to the nylon strap that goes under the shoe and is also held in place with a Velcro strip. An extra pair of straps is included with each pair of gaiters. These gaiters can also be worn with many of the low-top hiking boots either as is or by lengthening the strap. **Western States 100-Mile Endurance Run, www.ws100.com**

Lacing Options

Some runners have problems with laces causing friction and pressure. After a long run or hike, some runners and hikers experience bruising over the instep where the laces tie. Laces can be adjusted to fine-tune the fit of the shoe or boot and to relieve pressure over the instep. The lacing variations described below can make a shoe fit better and allow for needed spacing in the tongue area or provide for better heel control. The conventional method of lacing—crisscross to the top of the shoe—works best for the majority of people. But in some cases, other lacing patterns may alleviate trouble arising from the shape of a foot or the construction of the shoe. In the illustrations below, dotted lines show where laces are hidden from view.

Other than changing your lacing patterns, you might consider several lacing products that work well for running shoes, some boots, and many types of shoe. Easy Laces have been around for over 20 years and are a favorite with many athletes. These products replace the normal shoelaces and end the problem of laces coming untied or breaking. Experiment with stretch laces to find the most comfortable degree of lace tightness that does not cause undue pressure on the instep and yet controls the heel. A tongue cushion can help with instep irritations.

Lacing Tips

To prevent laces from untying, don't double-knot at the top. Instead, gather the loops and lace ends and tuck them through one or two of the cross-strands toward the toe of the shoe. This prevents laces from coming untied as effectively as double-knotting and is easier to untie. Also, when you're running through brush it keeps the laces from getting snagged or picking up debris.

Physician's assistant and ultrarunner Rich Schink suggests another method for keeping laces tied. First, make your laces as short as possible so the loops are not too long. Then add a simple knot at the ends of each lace. When tying your shoes, instead of leaving extra lace, pull on each of the loops until each end knot is snug to the bow. Finally, tuck the loops under one or two of the lace crossings.

Ian's Shoelace Site (**www.fieggen.com/shoelace/index/htm**) describes and shows a variety of knots for tying shoes. Ian's Secure Shoelace Knot is the best for active athletes.

If you will be in wet or cold weather, steer clear of loosely woven or cotton laces. Check your local outdoor store for laces made of polyester, nylon, or a blend of materials. Many athletes find their round laces come untied faster than any other design. Kevlar laces are very strong but may have to be double-knotted to stay tied.

Tying the laces too tightly can create pressure on the bony, thin-skinned tops of your feet. This can be worse if you have high arches or your shoes have thin tongues. Try flat instead of round laces, use one of the elastic laces below, or lace your shoes according to the foot-appropriate pain illustration (see below).

Lacing Methods

Flat feet, high arches or not enough support in the arches, narrow or wide feet, and heel-control problems can be helped, to varying degrees, by lacing techniques. Several of the lacing techniques described below work best with shoes having alternating eyelets spaced in a zigzag pattern, rather than in a straight line.

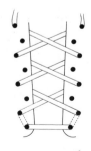

Lacing pattern for narrow feet.

For Narrow Feet

For narrow feet, use the eyelets farthest from the tongue of the shoe. This will bring up the sides of the shoe for a tighter fit across the top of the foot. This method works on shoes with variable-width eyelets.

For Wide Feet

For wide feet, use the eyelets closest to the tongue of the shoe. This gives the foot more space by leaving more width across the lace area. This method works best on shoes with variable-width eyelets. An alternative method is to pass back under the lace as it emerges from the second eyelet. This prevents the lace across the first eyelets from getting tighter as you run.

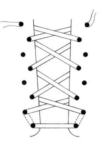

Lacing pattern for
wide feet.

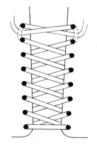

Lacing pattern to
prevent heel slippage.

To Prevent Heel Slippage

For hell slippage or heel problems, use every eyelet, making sure that the area closest to the heel is tied tightly and that the area nearer the toes has less tension. When you have reached the next to the last eyelet on each side, thread the lace through the top eyelet of the same side, leaving a small arch of lace between the eyelets. Then thread the opposite lace through each opposite arch before tying the laces together at the top.

For High Arches

For high arches, lace the shoes so the laces go straight across. After lacing the bottom two eyelets on the outer side to the inner two eyelets, lace up two eyelets on the same inner side and cross over to the outer side. Lace through these two eyelets and move up two eyelets on the same outer side.

Continue this alternating method until one set of eyelets is left. Continue lacing up to the top eyelets on each side.

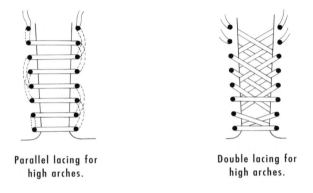

Parallel lacing for
high arches.

Double lacing for
high arches.

A high-arch lacing alternative is to string one lace through the first two bottom eyelets and then every other eyelet to the top. A second lace is threaded through the remaining eyelets. This allows tighter lacing at the ball of the foot and the ankle while the midfoot is laced looser. With this method, quick adjustments are easily made for uphills and downhills.

For Narrow Heel & Wide Forefoot

For a narrow heel and wide forefoot, use two laces per shoe. Lace one through the bottom half of the eyelets tied loosely. Lace the other through the top half of the eyelets tied more tightly than the bottom lace. Another

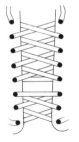

Lacing pattern for narrow
heel & wide forefoot.

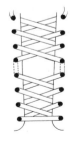

Avoid lacing over
the painful area.

option is to lace the first few loops loosely, tie a knot, and then lace the rest of the way up the shoe.

For Foot Pain

To alleviate foot pain, lace as normal for your foot type but skip the eyelets over the area of pain.

For Toenail Problems or Corns

For toenail problems or corns, lace down from the top eyelet opposite the problem toe to the bottom eyelet on the side of the problem toe, leaving enough end to tie the laces together. Then lace from the bottom up, side to side until the top eyelet is reached. This method creates an upward tension on the bottom eyelet over the problem toe, relieving pressure.

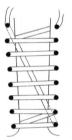

Alleviate pain caused by
toenail trouble or corns.

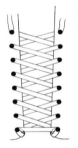

Locking the lace maintains
constant pressure at the toes.

For Constant Toe Pressure

To maintain constant pressure at the toes, lace the bottom eyelets as usual. Then lock the lace in place by looping the lace around and back through the same eyelet. Continue lacing as normal. Locking the lace at the second or third eyelet can modify this technique. This allows you to tie the laces as tight as you want above the lock while keeping the laces as loose as desired below the lock.

LACE PRODUCTS

EASY LACES are lockable shoelaces featuring a stretchy elastic cord with a lock where the usual bow is tied. You can slip your foot into the shoe or boot without releasing the lock, or you can release the lock to open the shoe further. The laces are available in a myriad of colors. For those not wanting the lock at the instep, cross the right lace over and under the shoe and through the lock. This moves the lock to the side of the shoe. **Stretch-Lace Co., (800) 572-3247, www.easy-lace.com**

HAPAD TONGUE CUSHIONS prevent rubbing and alleviate other irritations at the instep. If you have narrow heels, they also hold the foot back into the heel of the shoe for a better fit. The coiled, springlike wool fibers provide firm and resilient support. The pad attaches to the underside of the tongue of the shoe. **Hapad Inc., (800) 544-2723, www.hapad.com**

LACELOCKS, sometimes called cordlocks, are simple plastic cylinders with a button that locks or releases a lace run through a center hole. Two laces easily fit through the hole, which secures the laces at the desired tension. These are usually found in sporting goods stores.

THE LACE-STICK is for athletes whose laces come untied. Offered in a small tube, Lace-Stick is a sticky, waxlike, invisible, and safe substance. Use it to coat laces to prevent them from untying. **Idea to Sales, www.lacestick.com**

LOCK-LACES feature specially designed elastic laces combined with a spring-activated locking device. The high-tension springs are made from a metal alloy that won't rust or corrode. The locking device holds the laces (when knotted) in place so they stay secure and maintain the same constant tension on the foot. Available in a variety of colors and lengths. **Street Smart, LLC, (877) 445-2237, www.locklaces.com**

THE SHOELACE PLACE offers a wide variety of laces in assorted colors and lengths. They give a description of the laces including what the laces are made of. **Message/fax (513) 821-1716, www.lacesforless.com**

SPEED LACES consist of six plastic eyelet fittings, laces, a cord-lock, and a lace-pull. The risers fasten into the lace holes and allow the laces to tighten evenly above the surface of the shoes. The cord-locks and lace-pulls allow self-adjusting equal tension of the laces. **Speed Laces, (800) 880-3427, www.speedlaces.com**

LACE PRODUCTS

ULTIMATE SHOELACES are unique elastic laces with small, soft, collapsible knots about every half inch. This unique lace allows different tensions between eyelets of the same shoe. When you stretch the lace, the knots disappear. Simply stretch the laces to feed them through the eyelets of your shoes. After lacing, adjust the tension between eyelets. The ProKnot Ultimate Sport Lace has a 2:1 stretch ratio, and the PowerKnot Ultimate Extreme Lace has a 5:1 ratio. Laces come in a variety of colors and lengths. **Quest Technologies, Inc., (866) 566-8926, www.theultimateshoelace.com**

The **YANKZ SURE LACE SYSTEM** includes expandable cord laces and locking devices with two points of adjustability, providing a custom fit. A toe-clip hook holds the extra loop of lace. Shoes can be changed without unlocking the laces. **Yankz, (877) 892-6548, www.yankz.com**

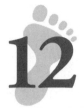

Self Care for Your Feet

Skin Care

In order to keep our feet healthy, it is necessary to take care of them, and that includes giving them the attention they need. But then how many of us know what our feet really need? Jillian Standish, a certified massage therapist, feels many runners simply don't think about using lotions or creams on their feet.

In the summer when we are most active, our feet are often abused. They become hard and callused or blistered by our multiday hikes, long training runs on back-to-back days, cross-sport training, going barefoot, or wearing sandals without socks. We repeatedly stress our feet without giving them time to recover and heal. In dry and cold weather our skin becomes dry, resulting in cracks in the skin. When these cracks are deep, they are called *fissures* and are often accompanied by calluses.

Use creams or lotions that help improve the skin's texture and tone by exfoliating dry and dead skin and allowing newly rejuvenated skin to emerge. Some creams contain alpha hydroxy acids, which are all-natural substances found in fruits and sugar cane that generally speed up the exfoliation process.

The use of a deep-penetrating hydrating cream twice a day will help your feet stay soft and supple by restoring your feet's natural oils. Ultrarunner

Roy Pirrung uses flaxseed oil products to keep his skin well conditioned. Pay close attention to your heels and the balls of your feet, two of the places where fissures and calluses typically form. To help the cream work its magic, at bedtime rub in the cream and place plastic wrap over your heels. The wrap seals in the cream to enhance the moisturizing effect. In the morning after showering, use a pumice stone or callus file to buff the skin and reduce calluses. After this buffing, rub in a small amount of cream to keep them soft during the day.

A good testimonial for soft feet comes from race walker Dave Littlehales:

> I used to think that tough, callused feet were the way to go. But after the '97 Vermont 100, where I developed huge full-bottom-of-the-feet blisters bilaterally, my podiatrist convinced me to go 100 percent in the other direction—soft and supple. Now I get a pedicure at least once a month, which smoothes out all calluses and rough spots. I also put creams on my feet on a daily basis. When I hit the trails or roads, I use foot powder. Things have improved greatly.

Keeping Feet Fresh

It's very easy to keep your feet and shoes fresh by using a small amount of baking soda. Use it as a powder on your feet or sprinkle a bit into your shoes to control odor. A short spray of Lysol into each shoe is another option to help control odor.

Long-distance hiker Brick Robbins finds that after several months on the trail he has a hard time with "stuff" growing on his feet. He has solved this common problem by soaking his feet for 20 minutes in a solution of about a gallon of water and 2 to 4 ounces of provi-done-iodine every week or so. It has kept his "feet from smelling too bad and seemed to kill the stuff that had started to grow under one of my big toes." Betadine can be used as an alternative to providone-iodine.

If your shoes get stinky or have a mildew smell after getting soaked in rain, wash them with soap and water and let them dry naturally. After they have dried, give each shoe a couple shots of Lysol. Do not put your shoes in the dryer.

SKIN PRODUCTS

FOOTSMART carries a complete line of skin-care products made for the feet. Total Foot Recovery Cream comes in three formulas: Original, Tree Tea Oil, and Shea Butter. Callus Treatment Cream with Urethin breaks down painful, hardened skin. Callex Callus Ointment and the Credo Callus Rasp reduce thick calluses. **FootSmart Products, (800) 870-7149, www.footsmart.com**

ZIM'S CRACK CREAM helps to moisturize, soothe, and soften dry, cracked, painful skin. You can choose between two formulas: a nighttime liquid or daytime cream. The creams are formulated with their unique herbal base of arnica and myrcia oil. **Perfecta Products, (800) 319-2225, www.crackcream.com**

By the end of summer many athletes are suffering from dry and cracked feet—usually from going barefoot or wearing sandals. If you have not had success with your current choice of foot lotion or cream, try Vicks VapoRub. Larry E. Millikan, M.D., a professor of dermatology at the Tulane University School of Medicine, says the petroleum in VapoRub holds in moisture, may have antifungal properties, and can reduce itching. A wide assortment of skin products that are useful for athletes is readily available at your local health food store or drugstore, including the following:

- Aquaphor Healing Ointment, for dry, cracked, blistered skin and chapped lips.
- Burt's Bees Coconut Foot Cream.
- Dr. Scholl's Ultra Overnight Foot Cream and Rough Skin Removing Foot Cream.
- Flaxseed oil products containing sources of essential fatty acids for proper skin conditioning.
- FootTherapy Natural Mineral Foot Bath for soaking and softening corns and calluses.

- Johnson's No More Rash, a unique 3-in-1 formula that promotes effective healing, soothes red, irritated skin, and forms a protective barrier. Contains zinc oxide and skin conditioners such as lanolin, petrolatum, and vitamins E and B5.
- Neutrogena Foot Cream, a Norwegian formula that moisturizes and softens dry skin.
- Pretty Feet & Hands Ultra Moisturizing Cream and Pretty Feet & Hands Rough Skin Remover, made by B.F. Ascher & Co. Pharmaceuticals.
- Vogel's Homeopathic 7 Herb Cream, a combination of herbs and oils in a natural base formulated to soften and smooth rough, dry, or cracked skin. Made by Bioforce of America.

Foot Massage

Massage is great for the feet. It helps increase circulation to injured areas and the increased blood supply helps speed recovery while reducing swelling. Sports massage focuses on releasing tight, contracted, over-worked muscles used in your sport or activity to restore them to their optimum condition.

Inflexibility associated with tightness can hinder efficient training and performance. When muscles are relaxed and receiving better circulation, they are stronger and tolerate higher levels of training with less pain and breakdown. Tight muscles can lead to strains and soft-tissue injury. Chronic tightness can cause muscle and connective tissue injury and inflammation, resulting in biomechanical imbalances, back pain, Achilles tendinitis, and plantar fasciitis. This is where massage and stretching can help.

Jillian Standish is a certified massage therapist whose typical clients are average athletes who need the benefits of massage to enhance their running. She devotes time during her massages to the feet since the lower leg muscles attach into the feet. As a pre-race conditioner, the massage helps loosen the muscles, often lengthening the runner's stride. As a post-race conditioner, she massages knots out of tired and stressed muscles.

Healing from many injuries can be speeded with massage. Mild strains can be eliminated with a few sessions of deep-tissue muscle massage. When a serious strain involves torn muscle fibers, scar tissue develops, which can cause pain when the muscle contracts. Stretching and joint movement combined with deep longitudinal massage strokes can help break down this scar tissue. Chronic tendinitis associated with scar tissue and adhesions in tendons may be resolved with sessions of deep cross-fiber friction massage. Some practitioners use active release techniques (ART) soft-tissue treatments. This treatment softens and stretches fibrous scar tissue, resulting in improved circulation, increased range of motion, and increased strength.

Look for a licensed massage therapist in the phone book, ask other athletes for referrals, or check your local sports stores for practitioners in your area. Likewise, physical therapists, sports-medicine chiropractors, and specialists in sports and orthopedic rehabilitation often incorporate massage into their practices.

Self-Massage

To do a self-massage of your feet, start by warming your feet in a bath or with warm, moist towels. Cross one leg over the other with the sole facing you. Use both thumbs to massage your feet in a deep, circular motion, working small areas at a time. Work from your toes toward your heel, and then to your ankle. Use various movements and pressure to find what feels best. All movement, and pressure, should be toward the heart—moving the old "stagnated" blood back to your heart. The use of massage oil or creams can help with the kneading of the skin and can soften dry heels and calluses. Self-foot massage is easier if you're limber, but even if you're not, you can manage it. If possible, have a partner to massage your feet.

Foot Massage Techniques

- Bottoms of your feet—Place your thumbs on the heel of one foot. Apply pressure to the underside of the foot starting at the bottom and slowly move towards the toes.
- Heels—Massage the bottom and sides of heel using your thumbs.
- Toes—Stroke between the toes upward toward the heart.

- Top of the foot—Using your fingers, massage the top of the foot focusing on the soft points between the bones of the forefoot upward towards the ankle.

- Stroking the foot—Using both hands, place your fingers on the top of the foot and the thumbs underneath. One hand at a time, stroke upward (slide your hands toward the ankle).

MASSAGE PRODUCTS

HAND & FOOT MASSAGE (2002) by Mary Atkinson also covers pedicures. ISBN 1842221663. **Carlton Books**

NATURAL FOOT CARE: HERBAL TREATMENTS, MASSAGE, AND EXERCISES FOR HEALTHY FEET (1998) by Stephanie Tourles presents a holistic approach to caring for feet, introducing alternative and natural treatments for good foot health. ISBN 1580170544. **Storey Books**

THE STICK is a massage tool that can be used on any major muscle groups through clothing or directly on the skin. It provides instant myofascial release that promotes healthy and relaxed muscle fibers and good circulation. It comes in four sizes and can be used before and after exercise to aid strength, flexibility, and endurance. **The Stick/RPI of Atlanta, (888) 882-0750, www.thestick.com**

Hydration, Dehydration & Sodium

A subject often overlooked by athletes is the effect on the skin of dehydration and the loss of important electrolytes. Long periods of physical exercise cause stress to the extremities as fluid accumulates in the hands and feet. Fingers and toes often swell as they retain fluid because of low blood sodium (hyponatremia). This causes foot problems as the soft, waterlogged tissues become vulnerable to the rubbing and pounding as we continue to run and hike.

Make sure that you replace electrolytes, especially on long events. Drinking water or even sports drinks may not provide the proper replacement of sodium and other important electrolytes. The popular energy bars and gels may also be low in the electrolytes needed by the body.

Karl King, developer of the SUCCEED! Buffer/Electrolyte Caps, points out that the maintenance of proper electrolyte levels will reduce swelling of hands and feet even after many hours of exercise, by reducing "hot spots" and blisters on the feet. "When there is heat and humidity, the sweat rate is high and sodium is usually lost in significant amounts," he says. "The sodium comes from the blood stream, and when the plasma gets too low, the

HYDRATION & ELECTROLYTES

E-CAPS ENDUROLYTES are formulated to counteract the effects of electrolyte depletion and imbalances of hot weather. The caps can be taken as a supplement or mixed in any fluid replacement drink. The Endurolyte caps contain calcium, magnesium, potassium, sodium chloride, L-tyrosine, vitamin B-6, and manganese. **E-CAPS Hammer Nutrition Ltd., (800) 336-1977, www.e-caps.com**

SUCCEED! BUFFER/ELECTROLYTE CAPS replenish in the proper proportions electrolytes commonly found in blood plasma, supporting hours of exercise. They are designed for individuals engaging in physical activities where they sweat heavily. The caps contain a chemical buffering system of sodium chloride, sodium bicarbonate, sodium citrate, sodium phosphate, and potassium chloride, which neutralizes the acids formed during heavy exercise. This both reduces nausea associated with exercise, particularly in the heat, and reduces the swelling of hands and feet common after many hours of exercise. Using the caps often leads to a reduction in hot spots and blisters. They should not be used when water is in short supply. **UltraFit, (888) 838-2802, www.ultrafit-endurance.com**

THERMOTABS are buffered salt tablets that can be taken to prevent muscle cramps or heat prostration due to excessive perspiration. The active ingredients are sodium chloride and potassium chloride. Look for Thermotabs at your local drugstore or pharmacy. **Menley & James Laboratories, Inc.**

body reacts to maintain the minimal tolerable level by pushing water from the blood into extracellular spaces. Thus, hands and feet swell. When the tissue on the feet swells, they become soft and more susceptible to blisters and damaged toenails." Many times the water that creates blisters is underneath the skin, not on the surface.

As ultrarunner Jay Hodde notes, "Proper hydration and well hydrated should not be used interchangeably. Being well hydrated with fluids says nothing about the sodium content of the fluid; both are important." When you are well hydrated yet have low sodium, extra fluid accumulates in the tissues of the feet and the likelihood of blister formation increases. When you become fluid-deficient, the skin loses its normal levels of water and in turn loses its turgor. Then it easily rubs or folds over on itself, which leads to blisters.

Many athletes have found out the hard way that simply drinking a fluid replacement drink often will not provide the necessary electrolytes in the proper concentrations that the body needs. The use of a sodium replacement product in prolonged physical activity can help in the prevention of blisters.

Changing Your Shoes & Socks

Whether you are close to an age-group win, a personal best, simply finishing within the time limit, or reaching a specific trail destination, the 3 to 10 minutes necessary for foot care may seem like a lifetime. Only you can make the decision on taking the time to care for your feet. I have seen many runners take off their shoes and socks to reveal skin that falls off the bottoms—not small pieces but enough to cover half their foot! It cannot be emphasized enough—take the time necessary to manage your feet or they will manage you.

When possible, change your shoes and socks before problems develop. You may opt to carry an extra pair of socks and a small foot-care kit in a fanny pack, allowing for road or trailside foot care as necessary. Dry skin is more resistant to blister formation than skin that has been softened by moisture. Depending on the event, you may choose to change at predetermined points or predetermined times. At these times, you should inspect your feet for problems and treat them appropriately. Power and/or lubricants should be reapplied when changing socks.

For long runs, determine in advance how often you will change your shoes and socks. Ultrarunner Dave Scott changes his shoes four to five times in a 100-mile trail race. At each change he reapplies more Vaseline to his toes. Aid stations that are accessible to crew support or aid stations that have your drop bags are the best places to change shoes. On a 24-hour run having additional half- or full-size larger shoes available may save your feet.

Changing shoes can help tired feet become refreshed. Since cushioning and support is different in each style of shoe, your feet may feel better in changed shoes. Each shoe's fit and dynamics has the potential to alter your gait and bring relief to your feet, ankles, knees, hips, and back—but a change can cause problems, too. If you are changing shoes to get rid of a hot spot, be aware that sometimes relief new shoes bring to one area can result in other problems elsewhere. Simply pay close attention to your feet as you start out in your changed shoes. Sometimes it is necessary to go back to the old shoes.

TIP: Horning In

Whenever you change shoes and/or socks, be sure to smooth your socks to avoid problem-producing wrinkles. Run your hand inside the shoe to smooth the shoe's seams and check for any irritating debris. When changing socks or shoes, too many athletes simply shove their feet into their shoes. This puts pressure on the heels and tender skin. Use a shoehorn when changing shoes to ease sore feet back into the shoe. The shoehorn will also help keep intact any taping you may have done to your feet. If you have an untaped blister on your heel, the pressure can tear the skin off the blister. Plan ahead and add an inexpensive shoehorn into each drop bag or aid station foot-care kits.

Trail running and hiking often make for wet shoes and boots that become dirt-caked. Change shoes and socks as soon as possible after getting wet. Even though shoes and socks do dry out after a stream crossing or in rain, continuing to run or hike may cause the skin on your feet to become overly soft and tender and more prone to blisters. Softening of the skin, called

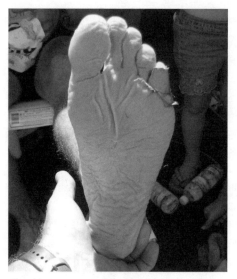

The skin creases on this severely macerated foot resulted from not changing shoes and socks.

maceration, can cause skin over and around blisters to separate. Where the blister is already ruptured, the skin then opens up. When the skin has been wet for long periods of time, it is not uncommon, when removing socks, to find the skin as shriveled as a prune and the skin separating. The use of high-technology oversocks (see page XX in the chapter on socks) to keep the feet dry can help reduce maceration and blisters.

Hikers need to carry a basic foot-care kit as part of a first-aid kit. They should wash their dirty socks daily and dry them on the back of their packs. Some hikers will wisely choose to change socks several times a day. If possible, take a few minutes for a short 5 to 10 minutes' soak in a cold stream or lake to refresh your tired feet. Before putting stream washed socks back on your feet, turn them inside out and fluff up the fabric to restore some of their loft.

In extremely cold weather, it is important to keep feet dry and warm. Socks and footwear that are too tight can cause constriction and impede circulation. Changing from wet into dry socks helps keep the feet warm. The use of moisture-wicking socks also is helpful. See the section on high-technology oversocks (page 78) for information on how these socks can help ward off cold.

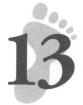

Extreme Conditions & Multiday Events

Cold and wet, frostbite, heat, jungle rot, sand, snow and ice, trench foot, and multiday events are conditions that adventure racers, ultra-runners, and travelers need to understand. The interesting thing is that many of these conditions can be experienced in the same event.

During the ELF Adventure Race, Steve Guerny's team had to deal with many foot-care issues: hotspots, blisters, grit, water, swelling, water, jungle rot, water—all common elements in a multiday adventure race. Some sports test and challenge us in different environments. These events will also challenge your foot-care skills. Because of the uniqueness of each event, there are tips that will work in one environment and not in another.

personal experience

I'm convinced one of the key factors in [our success] was conscientious foot care. We realized that with such a wet course, damaged feet were to be the telling factor. We actually learned from the horse-riding stage—gee, if the horses are having problems with their feet, we will have it worse. It was exceptionally wet.

"Our simple strategy was to keep our feet as dry and undamaged as possible. Prevention is infinitely better than cure, but be efficient about it. At every rest or stop, we made sure we immediately dropped to the ground and elevated our feet to reduce swelling. If the stop was a long one (more than 60 seconds), we took our shoes off and allowed our feet to dry. This was especially effective in the sun. The heat helped to dry and the UV killed some bugs.

"Cleanliness was important, and as I started to get jungle rot, I used copious quantities of that magic Betadine. We cleared grit out frequently but quickly. Several times our feet started to swell to the point that we could feel damage occurring, so we stopped to allow the swelling go down. When we did move, we moved quickly and efficiently so as to reduce time on feet.

"I used insoles that molded to my feet and shoes, which also helped to reduce blisters, and they proved easy to modify with a knife to relieve hotspots. Several teammates used SealSkinz socks to keep the grit and infection out. We used a silicon lubricant to attempt to seal out moisture and to lubricate. I guess the ultimate key is to thoughtfully think about the conditions and plan smart."

—Steve Guerny, on winning the ELF Adventure Race

Jane Moorhead worked on participants' feet at the 2003 Primal Quest Adventure Race. Her experiences second Steve Guerny's points about planning for foot care under various conditions.

personal experience

"In the day I worked we saw almost 20 racers. Close to 75 percent of them had at least some degree of immersion foot, and they all had blisters in various stages. One racer told me that he had taken three pairs of socks and changed them religiously when his feet got wet. Another team cut the toes out of their $90 shoes in order to promote draining. Most of them had applied tape, moleskin, or some other type of dressing.

"So why were their feet in such bad condition? My husband worked the race as the support team leader for an Australian team. Out of the four people on his team, two had badly macerated tissue from broken blisters on the balls of their feet and two did not. Why? I wish I had an absolute answer, but I think there are many factors.

"Keeping feet dry is a must. One racer had such bad immersion foot that when he removed the tape from the bottom of his foot, he took a couple of layers of skin with it. We began turning people away from the tent until they had washed and dried their feet and let them bake in the sun awhile to dry the tissues out. The best taping in the world wasn't going to work on wet feet.

"*Know your feet!* Those who had used taping or moleskin going into the event fared better than those who didn't. If a racer knows that he or she tends to get pinch blisters on their little toes, they need to tape at the start of the race, not during.

"Racers should stop at the first sign of foot trouble to tape their feet. This was a demanding race, so even the most experienced racers may have underestimated the toll it would take on their feet. However, my impression was that many teams just wanted to keep moving and didn't take the necessary 10 minutes to tape.

"And finally, sometimes you are just blessed with tough feet. Sorry, but it's true."

—Jane Moorhead,
after working on feet at the 2003 Primal Quest Adventure Race

Never assume that you are blessed with such tough feet. Use the following tips based on the event's location, weather, terrain, length, and how your feet have held up in past events. Read the whole section on multiday events, since extreme and multiday events are often related.

Cold & Wet

At one time or another, every one of us has trained or competed in an event in which our feet were cold and wet for long periods of time. In a short event, these conditions could persist for a couple of hours. In a one-day event, they could last four to eight hours, and in a long event they may last four to eight hours a day for continuous days. However long the period, this wet condition can have a negative effect on our feet. Blisters may go from being minor inconveniences to major problems. Maceration can happen. In severe cases, trench foot can become a real medical issue. When these conditions set in, you will be at the mercy of your hurting feet.

Wet and cold feet can lead to long-term and even permanent disability. Even at temperatures above freezing, the combination of cold and moisture can lead to serious injury. Trench foot can occur even in mid 60-degree temperatures in such activities as backpacking. The care of your feet in cold weather is crucial in many sports.

Rich Schick, an ultrarunner and physician's assistant, gives important advice about being cold:

> The first thing to remember is that at any level of activity you only have a limited total amount of heat produced by the body. The body is going to give priority to the vital organs and only send what is left over out to the hands and feet. This is why the first step to keeping the feet warm is to make sure that the torso and especially the head and neck are kept warm. Likewise, if the legs are bare or inadequately protected, a lot of heat will be lost before it ever reaches the feet. Next, you must understand the principal of how insulation works. Clothing traps air and allows the body to heat it. If insulation is compressed, it is no longer insulation. In the feet this translates to you can't have tight footgear and expect your feet to stay warm.

Rich identifies a key problem: "Feet either get wet from environmental conditions of rain or snow or as a result of wet snow or especially slush on the ground. Terrain factors of stream crossing and standing water also are sources of wet feet. Surprisingly, the most common cause of wet feet is the enemy within, perspiration. This combination of factors usually makes the reality of the situation a matter of how to deal with wet feet rather than how to keep your feet dry."

So what happens when your feet are wet and cold and how can that affect your racing? As your skin becomes wet, it softens and becomes more susceptible to blisters. If a blister forms, it is more likely to rupture. The skin then separates further. Maceration happens when skin becomes soft and wet for long periods of time. When you take off your socks and find your feet look like prunes, this is what has happened. The skin is tender and can fold over on itself, separating and creating problems. As layers of skin separate, blisters spread, the skin becomes whitish in color, and it can split open and bleed. It is very hard to patch feet when this has happened. Feet become so tender that every step is painful.

Again, Rich offers good advice: "You must protect the feet from maceration or skin breakdown. A light coat of Vaseline or other petroleum jelly is inexpensive and quite effective. I find that a beeswax and lanolin preparation such as Kiwi's Camp Dry is even more effective. It is

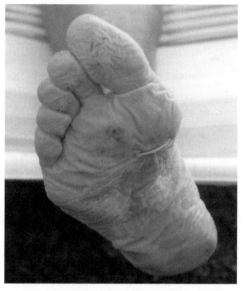

A macerated foot resulting from exposure to moisture.

designed to waterproof footgear but has more durability than the Vaseline-type products. For those with especially sweaty feet, a quick spray with an antiperspirant prior to the application of the barrier ointment can be very helpful." Another good choice is Hydropel Sports Ointment, which is used by many adventure racers because of its moisture-repelling capabilities.

Many athletes with macerated feet feel as if the whole bottom of their foot is blistered. In fact, there are often no blisters. The skin is so soft and tender that every step is painful. These feet need to be dried as much as possible by removing them from the moisture source, applying drying powders, and exposing them to air. On occasion I have used a large 3-inch 2nd Skin circle over the ball of the foot in an attempt to relieve the pain. But there is no quick fix for macerated feet.

Tips for Managing Cold & Moisture

Consider the following pointers when planning any training or competitive event in which cold and moisture will be an issue:

- For high-intensity, fast-paced sports, lightweight and fast-drying shoes are the best bet.

- If your shoes have a breathable upper, a layer of duct tape over the upper can keep the wind and moisture out.

- Wearing shoes that do not have adequate draining capabilities will subject your feet to extended periods of moisture. Use a heated nail or a drill to make a few small holes where your upper attaches to the lower part of your shoe or boot. Make one on each side of the heel and one on each side of the forefoot. Some athletes prefer holes in the sole of the shoe for faster draining.

- Wear socks that are have moisture-wicking capabilities. Choose synthetic fabrics such as CoolMax or Olefin or a blend of materials. SmartWool socks, made from wool, are good in wet conditions. Whatever socks you wear, change them frequently and dry the old socks.

- Consider wearing waterproof socks. You have two choices. The SealSkinz WaterBlocker and ChillBlocker socks are designed to keep water out. The Seirus Neo-Sock or StormSock are made from neoprene and are designed to hold warmth in, but some water can get inside. Even with these socks if your feet get wet from sweat, they will still suffer, albeit to a lesser degree.

- Some recommend using a plastic bag over your socks or between two pairs of socks. While this can keep your feet from getting soaked, your feet will get wet from sweat.

- Foot powders that absorb moisture can help keep your feet dry. Put small containers of powder into your drop bags and in your pack. Reapply powder when changing socks. Zeasorb or Odor-Eaters both make a good moisture-absorbing powder that does not cake up into clumps. Wipe off the old powder and grit before applying new powder.

- When resting or sleeping, take off your wet shoes and socks to allow your feet to breathe.

Trench Foot

The name "trench foot" originated during World War I, when the troops stood in cold, wet trenches for days without relief. It is sometimes called "immersion foot."

Trench foot is a serious nonfreezing cold injury that develops when the skin of the feet is exposed to a combination of moisture and cold for extended periods. Tissue death can occur in feet exposed to moisture and cold in boots or shoes that constrict the feet for periods of 12 hours or longer. It can occur in temperatures as high as 60 degrees if the feet are constantly wet—in other words, it does not have to be in winter conditions.

Trench foot is caused by factors common to athletes participating in extreme sports: dehydration, wet shoes and socks, poor nutrition, inadequate and too tight footwear, and cold. Many of the multiday ultramarathons and adventure races can create conditions right for trench foot. Under the right conditions, even a one-day event could jeopardize your feet. Similarly, hikers can find themselves in the same conditions.

Due to the cold, wet, and constricting environment inside the shoe, vasoconstriction (blood vessels constricting) reduces circulation to preserve heat loss. With the resulting lack of oxygen and nutrients in the blood, toxins build up and skin tissue begins to die. The skin reddens and becomes numb. Swelling follows with associated itching and tingling pain. When the skin rewarms, blisters form, and when they fall off, ulcers develop, and then open and weep or bleed. If trench foot is left untreated, amputation may be required.

Remember it can take 24 to 48 hours before the severity of the damage is fully apparent. If your feet are painful and swollen, and develop blisters, you need medical attention.

Tips for Avoiding Trench Foot

Trench foot is caused by factors common to athletes participating in extreme sports: dehydration, wet shoes and socks, poor nutrition, inadequate and too tight footwear, and cold. There are specific ways to reduce your chance of getting trench foot:

- Wash and dry your feet.

- Do not sleep in wet socks.

- Avoid socks and shoes that are too tight.

- Do not add socks if your feet are cold. This causes more constriction inside your shoes. Move up to a larger shoe.

- Rewarm gently; do not use a strong heat source.

- Do not rub the skin; instead, use passive skin-to-skin contact.

- Elevate the feet above the level of the heart.

- Start an anti-inflammatory drug program.

- Consider the use of an antiperspirant with aluminum hydroxide to reduce sweating—use this on your feet for a week before anticipated exposure.

- Do not pop blisters, apply lotions or creams, or walk on injured feet.

Frostbite

Frostbite occurs when tissue actually freezes. Toes are particularly susceptible to this serious condition. Factors that contribute to frostbite include exposure to wind, wet skin (even from sweat), and tight socks and shoes.

Early signs of frostbite include numbness, a waxy or pale discoloration of the skin, the tissue becoming firm to the touch, and pain in the area. As the frostbite progresses, the skin gets paler and the pain ceases. Often frostbite will thaw on its own as the person keeps moving or gets into a warm environment and out of the wind, wet, and cold. As the tissue warms, there can be redness, itching, and swelling.

In severe cases of frostbite, the skin becomes immobile as it freezes with underlying tissue. Blisters can form with clear or milky fluid. Blisters filled with blood indicate deeper damage. While the skin may change color, or even darken, do not assume you will lose the toes. It may take weeks or months to know if amputation is necessary. Check with your physician as soon as possible to determine what care is necessary.

Tips for Managing Frostbite

- Do not rub your toes to warm them—that causes even more tissue damage.

- Do not rub the frostbitten area.

- Unless absolutely necessary, don't allow the person to walk on frostbitten feet or toes.

- Get the person into a warm environment as soon as possible.

- Immerse the affected area in lukewarm—not hot—water, or warm the affected area with the body heat from another person.

- Do not use a heating pad, heat lamp, or the heat of a stove, fireplace, or radiator for warming.

- Do not rewarm or thaw a person's frostbite unless you are sure you can keep them warm. It is important to remember that thawing the tissue and then allowing it to refreeze can be devastating.

- Dehydration will make you more susceptible to frostbite.

Snow & Ice

Hiking or running on snow and ice can be challenging. Traction is often severely compromised and unless one is careful, falls are common. Snow can cover a variety of rocks, roots, and other obstacles that can cause you to trip. Ice is a hard and unforgiving surface. The two most important factors in traveling over snow and ice are keeping your feet relatively warm and obtaining dry traction.

Moisture-wicking socks are a must. Also consider wearing waterproof socks. You have two choices in these: the SealSkinz ChillBlocker socks, which have a fleece liner and will keep snow out; and the Seirus Neo-Sock or StormSock, which are made from neoprene and designed to hold warmth. These socks are described in the chapter on Socks (page 76).

Cole Hanley runs with hex screws in the soles of his shoes during the winter and has been pleased with the traction they provide. He adds that no screws have ever fallen out and no screws have ever poked the bottom of his feet. An alternative is to use one of the traction devices that fit over the soles of the shoes.

TIP: Hex Screws for Ice & Snow

Sheet-metal hex screws can be used in the soles of your shoes to get better traction. This is a cheap and easy way to modify your shoes or boots to be safe in snow and ice. Use $3/8$-inch screws in the lugs of your shoes' soles. Put 10 to 18 of them around the edges of your shoes with several at the toes and heels. Be careful if your shoes have an air or gel insert. Use a ratchet screwdriver or a drill with a $1/4$-inch socket to make the job easier. Dipping the screws into epoxy before screwing them into the shoes will help them stay in place.

Shoe companies are introducing shoes that incorporate some form of spikes for traction. Be on the lookout for these and similar shoes. North Face is marketing their Switchback shoe as "the most technically advanced trail running/adventure shoe ever created." In the sole of the shoe are six CHAMP Q-Lok spikes. These interchangeable spikes ensure maximum traction control on the road, trail, in heavy mud, ice, and snow. The spikes work with an aggressive sole design. Two spikes are offered, a soft spike and a Scorpion spike for use in extreme conditions. The shoes use the scree gaiter attachment and offer a two-tier lacing system that accommodates changes in your feet during multiday events. Check out the shoes at **www.thenorthface.com**.

The Icebug is a shoe and boot line from a Swedish footwear company. Their shoes have 16 "smart" studs that grip. The carbide-tip steel studs are set in the hefty rubber lugs on the shoe's sole. Four varieties of shoes and boots are offered. The Multi-Run version has six different models. Icebug shoes can be seen at **www.icebug.se**.

Tips for Managing Snow & Ice

■ Consider wearing one of the newer Gore-Tex fabric shoes to repel some of the moisture that will lead to wet and cold feet.

- Use sheet-metal hex screws or one of the traction devices listed below.
- Use gaiters to keep the snow out of your shoes or boots.
- Wear the best moisture-wicking sock available. Wool blend socks are a good choice.

WINTER TRACTION PRODUCTS

THE KAHTOOLA TRACTION SYSTEM, a flexible traction system, is designed to be used with any common footwear from trail-running shoes or hiking boots to snow boots. Kahtoola's 10-point gripping system is made from the strongest aluminum alloy and weighs only 19 ounces per pair. Straps and quick-release buckles make it easy to put the system on any shoe. A unique LeafSpring extender bar and independent front and rear straps allow the system to flex naturally with any footwear. The extender bar is available in three different lengths and can be adjusted easily without tools. **Kahtoola Inc., (866) 330-8030, www.kahtoola.com**

KASTNER TRACKTION SOLES were designed by Sid Kastner, a world-class triathlete. The Tracktion Sole's out sole has patented carbide-metal studs that extend slightly from rubber protrusions on the sole. When used for running in adverse conditions, these studs remain extended on snow, ice, or trail surfaces. On hard (concrete, asphalt) surfaces they are absorbed into the sole, so that they perform like any other high-performance running shoe. Presently, the Tracktion Sole is available for license to shoe manufacturers. **Kastner Shoe, (800) 811-7155, www.kastnershoe.com**

STABILICER SPORTS are traction devices that have an aggressive cleat-and-tread combination held in place with their tension-fit binding. They are made with dual-density TPE elastomer construction with replaceable cleats. **(800) 782-2423, www.32north.com**

WINTER TRACTION PRODUCTS

SUREFOOT ICE JOGGERS are made of a rubberized material that stretches over your soles. A diamond pattern of spikes allow for more push-off and gripping action. The spikes are molded of a tough plastic that holds up to the toughest cold-weather conditions. These are offered by Roadrunner Sports and other online sources. **www.roadrunnersports.com**

TI-GRRRIP! is a package of super-hard corundum particles and an adhesive to glue them to the soles of your shoes. Corundum, the third most prevalent mineral in the earth's crust, it is very hard (the second hardest mineral next to diamond), tough, and most importantly, natural to the environment. **Old Shoes, (303) 733-3211, www.shoetread.com**

YAKTRAX PRO is a lightweight traction device, made of rubber tubing covered with stainless steel coils, that fits across the soles of your shoes. The Pro is made out of an injection-molded thermal plastic elastomer designed for easy on and off. The coils are protected against rusting and hand-wound to give you 360 degrees of traction on ice and snow. The Pro is equipped with a removable performance strap that fits across the top of the shoe for stability. **Yaktrax, (866) 925-8729, www.yaktrax.com**

Heat

Heat can affect your feet when running on roads, like at the Death Valley Badwater Ultramarathon, or in the desert. We can learn from athletes who have been there. Cathy Tibbetts-Witkes, who has raced at Death Valley, the hottest place in America, describes running in the extreme heat:

> Unless you train [in the desert heat] your feet just aren't going to get used to pavement that you can cook fajitas on. With temperatures best measured with a meat thermometer, runners attempting Badwater have to figure out how to make their feet last 135 miles (bad enough as it is) in almost that much heat. Not only will your feet sweat, but also your crew will be spraying you with water to cool you down. As dry as the desert is, your feet will be wet at Badwater.

Five time Marathon des Sables finisher and 2002 Badwater finisher Blaise Supler was surprised at how few blisters she got at Badwater compared to the Marathon des Sables held in the desert of Morocco: "The pounding at Badwater killed me, especially on the downhill. Plus the skin on my feet turned white and soft, with creases, I guess from them being so wet. It made the soles of my feet seem like they were on fire." This fire sensation is caused by maceration of the feet, which is brought on when feet are wet over long periods. Supler admits that she "never changed my shoes or socks past mile 72. I was afraid to see my feet, they were so painful. But it turned out they were hardly blistered." Maceration is preventable by using moisture-wicking socks, changing them frequently, and allowing the feet to dry and the skin to return to normal.

Clive Saffery ran the extreme Badwater Ultramarathon from Death Valley to Mt. Whitney and came up with a creative method of protecting his feet from the heat. In the 1999 Badwater race, he added an extra precaution to his usual regimen of using of Vaseline and powder. To reduce heat on his feet, he duct-taped a cut-up space blanket on all the nonwhite parts of his shoe uppers and lined the under side of his shoe insoles in the same way, using small pieces of duct tape to hold the silver blanket on the shoe and insole. Aside from one small heel blister at 122 miles, he was trouble free the whole race in spite of the temperatures. The space blanket under his shoe insoles fared worse, however—when it was removed after the climb out of Death Valley, it had been reduced to a transparent piece of cling film! Some hot-water heater blankets are thin enough to be used the same way.

Probably no one has had the opportunity to work in the heat as much as Denise Jones. Her techniques have earned her the title of "Blister Queen" of Badwater.

"*personal experience*

The heat of the desert has melted shoes. Imagine what it does to feet! Over the past ten years I have seen and worked on feet so unbelievably blistered from this event it would make one think they have been boiled in oil. I have used a myriad of combinations to ensure that feet could handle the stresses of the Badwater

Ultramarathon. Through this trial-and-error method, I have devised a system of foot taping that seems to work specifically for racing on pavement in temperatures exceeding 120 degrees. It has been my experience that if I can get a runner to pretape, it helps prevent a lot of wasted time as the race progresses. Blistering, if it does occur, is subsequently not as major and more treatable.

"Try this method in training first to see if it works for you. In the 2003 race Ben's feet did perfect. In the horrific heat, he had no blisters. I used a combo of my taping, the Injinji socks, and Hydropel, as well as powder before placing his feet in the socks.

"I don't recommend duct tape. All tape should be breathable. This is very important in desert heat. We have found that duct tape doesn't breathe and causes the area that has been taped to become edematous, sometimes causing worse blisters underneath the tape.

"I have had no success using Blister Relief, formerly Compeed, for the heat. Some have used it to alleviate the pain of a blister quickly. The problem seems to be that it might help at the immediate time, but trying to get it off is a nightmare. It shifts on the skin and sticks so much it sometimes pulls the skin off, too."

—Denise Jones, the Badwater Blister Queen

Denise Jones's Tips for Controlling Foot Heat

- Pretape any potential problem areas on your feet. In the desert, a breathable tape is essential.
- Make sure the shoes aren't black, as they absorb heat.
- Wear moisture-wicking socks.
- The Injinji toe socks help protect each toe.
- Orthotics or extra insoles provide extra insulation from the heated pavement.
- Take several pair of shoes in larger sizes, so that if your feet swell in the event you can change to a larger size.
- You can also keep your shoes and socks cooler if you have room by placing them in Ziploc bags in the coolers.

- It's also a good idea to keep the tape in a Ziploc in your cooler, too, because the adhesive melts in the desert heat, even in the foot box. When it melts, it won't adhere to the foot.

- Have some substantial scissors available so if need be, you can cut your shoes in areas where friction has blistered you.

- Have a foot-care plan and the equipment to fix your feet.

Sand

It's all about the sand. Anyone who has traveled across sand knows how it gets into everything. Your goal is to keep it out of your shoes and socks. Take one race as an example: the Marathon des Sables (MdS), is a 150-mile race across the Sahara Desert of southern Morocco, which in which requires competitors to carry all their food and gear for the weeklong duration of the race.

Cathy Tibbetts-Witkes has done the MdS several times and has mastered the sand:

> With a little training, feet can get used to running long distances with a 15- to -20-pound pack. What your training at home can't replicate is the relentless sand, which commercially made gaiters don't sufficiently keep out. The trick to saving your feet at the MdS is to make your own gaiters, which completely cover your shoe and go up to your knee. I use 70- to 80-denier uncoated nylon and fasten them to my shoes with Velcro epoxied to the shoe.

Cathy's gaiters attach to the edge of the soles and end just below her knees (see photo of these gaiters on page 131).

Whether or not you wear gaiters, try to use shoes that are not mesh (unless you use gaiters like Cathy Tibbetts-Witkes). The mesh allows sand to get inside your shoes where it gets under your insoles, into your socks, and onto your feet. The sand, along with the movement of your feet inside the shoes, can tear up the shoes' inner material, causing even more irritations to your feet.

Jim Benike tells of what he learned about this event and the effects of the sand on his feet.

personal experience

"The Marathon des Sables is unique in that it lasts seven days so one has to run every day. One thinks in terms of sand, but there is so much grit and dust that is smaller than the sand. The grit will get into everything. Every crack and crevice—nothing escapes the grit. It will get into the mesh of any shoe. With that preface one can begin to discuss foot care.

"I used double-layer CoolMax socks, which I have been very satisfied with, but they are the wrong sock for this race. The grit and sand gets trapped between the two layers so after a day or two the socks turn into sandpaper. Hand washing will not remove the sand and grit. Plan on three pairs, which I think is the right number—one pair for the first three days, one for the long day, and one for the balance of the race.

"I wore gaiters every day. Aside from gaiters one needs to cover the mesh of the shoe for Dune day and the long day. I saw several versions of a full shoe gaiter, but they didn't seem to hold up. I tried duct tape on the toe box, but it fell off one shoe. I could have used more duct tape. I think nylon over the toe box might work—the grit would still get into the shoe, but at least heat could escape. Some people just used a large sock over the toe box.

"I wear size 12 shoes but ran in 13s with an extra shoe insole. I took the extra insole out after the second day because my feet were swelling as expected. I had sandals for after the race. My feet were almost too big. I saw several people who couldn't get their feet into shoes or sandals and walked around with shoe insoles duct-taped to their feet.

"The race is about blister prevention, then blister management. It is just a question of how soon the blisters start. I used New Skin on my blisters and potential blister areas. It made the skin tougher and didn't attract grit or sand. I also used duct tape over the ball of my feet, which is where I normally blister. Pretaping might have helped, but I didn't do it. I know of others, veterans of this event, who did pretape. The needle-and-thread method of draining blisters worked for me. I didn't have any infections. The air is so dry your feet fry out after each day's run. They never stay 'punky.'

"The French take the skin right off the top of the blister. In my opinion this is a bad idea because you still have to run the next day. A visit to the Medical tent was a sure sign of someone in deep trouble."

— Jim Benike on the Marathon des Sables

If you use a lubricant on your feet, watch for sand buildup on your toes and feet. The sand will stick to the lubricant and rub between your toes and feet, creating a course friction. When changing socks, wipe off any old lubricant and clean your feet before applying any new lube. Two-time MdS finisher Keith Baker recommends being "really careful with the sand and keeping your feet clean."

You may have noticed a theme in the advice from all these sand veterans: Sand can ruin your feet, and you need to do everything possible to keep it out of your shoes and socks.

Tips for Managing Sand

- Avoid shoes with mesh materials.
- Avoid double-layer socks.
- Keep your feet as clean as possible.
- Wipe off any old lubricant before applying a new coat.
- Use gaiters that keep the sand out of your shoes and socks.
- Stop and check your feet regularly.

Jungle Rot

Jungle rot is a skin disorder induced by a tropical climate. In long adventure races or ultramarathons, particularly in foreign countries, feet are often exposed to all sorts of organisms and nasty creatures. The ELF Adventure is one such race. It has been held in the Philippines and Brazil, places where a racer can be exposed to unfriendly parasites.

It's easy to pick up a few bugs—protozoa or mites or who knows what—especially when going through streams, rivers, and damp caves. Many of these parasites enter the skin through open blisters, cracks between the toes, fissures on the skin, and scratches. Some may lead to a hemorrhagic appearance under the skin. They may ooze fluid, often yellow with pus, from infection. The feet may be painful and itch unrelentingly. There are some nasty creatures out there in adventure racing, that's for sure!

In most cases, a diagnosis will have to be made by a physician and oral antibiotics prescribed. Some of these organisms will take weeks or months to be eliminated from your body. Many times the race organizations will be aware of the potential for this type of exposure and have medical recommendations for its control.

"H *personal experience*

aving experienced the worst foot problems I can imagine at the ELF, I can share what happened. What is it that allowed some teams to totally avoid foot problems while others had to quit? Should some of us spank our parents for bad genes or will enrolling in an Anthony Robbins firewalking course do the trick? My team took no special precautions and might be a good control group to help generate some ideas to prevent these problems for racers in similar environments in the future.

"Although the race's Website only listed three official withdrawals for 'sore feet,' it's likely feet played some part in many withdrawals. You could see many competitors hobbling. At one point my feet were swollen twice normal size with distention where there should have been arches. They had taken on a mottled white, blue, and pink coloring, and I'm told I probably had a fever due to the infections raging within.

"The doctors have told us that we experienced a combination of fungus and hookworms on top of the general blistering and swelling we had expected. The race conditions were very wet, and so were competitors' feet, from a combination of creek crossings and rain. Wet feet and fine grit led to blisters that in turn allowed penetration by the fungus under the skin, moving us from athlete's foot to Stay-Puff-Marshmallow feet. Subcutaneous fungal infections were the largest cause of pain and severe swelling. The doctor said hookworms are generally acquired in sandy soil that enters shoes and carries the organisms allowing them to burrow in. One teammate wore SealSkinz socks that kept the sand out and she didn't get hookworms. Those of us without SealSkinz were infected with the hookworms. I counted around thirty in my feet!

"Here is what little I learned. Betadine rocks. One of the French doctors suggested mixing Betadine with Vaseline, coating the feet, and wearing socks (and the obvious and ever so useless, 'Keep zee feet dry'). This really helped kill the external fungal infection as the stuff kills everything. Hookworms are easily treated by a single dosage of a prescription medicine that for me worked almost overnight.

"Hiking poles are a must for races this length, especially if there is any chance you may become foot impaired. I put 40 percent of my weight onto my Leki hiking poles for a good portion of the hiking sections and wouldn't have been capable of finishing without them."

— David Schmitt, who has raced in the ELF Adventure

Tips for Controlling Jungle Rot

- Do your utmost to keep your feet as dry as possible.

- Air them whenever possible, exposing them to sunlight when resting.

- Use a water-repelling ointment like Hydropel or Gurney Goo to keep moisture at bay.

- Change into dry clean socks as often as possible.

- When changing socks and shoes, check your feet for open skin and treat those areas with Betadine and an antiseptic ointment. Some lubricants are made with antibacterial properties. The "Compounds" chapter (page 90) lists several of these lubricants.

- If you suspect a parasite, get medically checked as soon as possible.

Foot Care in Multiday Events

Multiday events are a challenge to even the experienced athlete. There may be changing weather conditions; water from rain, wind and cold; and heat and humidity. No two multiday events will be the same. You must be prepared for whatever is thrown at you. Proper pre-event planning with your shoes, socks, and foot-care kit, along with your other gear, is crucial. Whether you are doing a 100-mile trail run that takes 40 hours, a six-day road race, a three-day adventure race, or a two-week backpack, you must take care of your feet from the start. Some suggestions are appropriate for road races but not for trail races or events that are a mix of road and trail. Modify the suggestions to fit your event.

Rob Byrne has participated in the Marathon des Sables in Morocco and the Gobi March in China, each a seven-day stage race about 150 miles in length. He uses Vaseline on his feet, and then a polypro liner sock and a cotton sock on top. Each day he gets a new pair of liner socks and replaces the cotton socks every other day. I cringe at his use of cotton socks, but they work for him. He had no blisters even with all the river crossings in the Gobi event. He does wear gaiters.

Adventure racer Ian Adamson gives three prerace tips for multiday events:

First, choose shoes that breathe and drain well. Water and moisture always get in, but you want to make sure they get out, and fast. Waterproof shoes have their place, but rarely on the feet of an ultra-endurance athlete since they have the propensity to turn your nicely conditioned feet to mush faster than you can say "hop, skip, and jump."

Second, look for adequate midsole cushioning. Racing flats are nice and light, but over a few days it will feel like you are walking with bare feet over the rocks. Too much cushioning is also bad since it elevates your feet, sacrificing lateral stability.

Third, some form of stone bruise protection is essential. The Salomon adventure racing shoes all have superior stone protection in the form of an outer sole Kevlar or plastic plate. Carrying extra weight in uneven, off-trail terrain can wreak havoc on the soft tissues of your feet with inadequate defense.

More Tips from Ian Adamson for Healthy Feet

Try a silicone-based lubricant, which helps drive moisture away from your skin and reduces friction between your feet and shoes. Sportslick and Hydropel are both good products.

Empty your socks of rocks and junk. The debris that accumulates as you thrash around in the forest can cause blisters, sores, abrasions, and cuts, all highly contraindicated for happy feet. Best of all, use a light gaiter to keep things out to start with.

Walk through very cold water whenever you can. This is extremely useful to reduce swelling and has some lovely, if painful, therapeutic and preventative effects while racing on your dogs. Don't worry about the moisture; if you have fast-draining shoes and use a silicone lubricant, you will be fine. Otherwise, soak your feet in whatever cold water is available.

Dan Brannen, an experienced multiday ultrarunner, has several ideas for the problem of swollen feet in multiday races:

> In the latter stages of multidays on tracks or road loops, my enlarging feet felt best with no socks and open-toe running shoes. The biggest cause of serious swelling during a multiday is, ironically, being off your feet. The best way to avoid really troublesome foot swelling is to stay on the track as much as possible. Any rest breaks longer than a few hours are just going to make your feet bigger. Forget icing, elevation, and rest during the race. Their effect will be inconsequential.

Dan also recommends, wearing sandals over socks when traveling home after the event (especially when flying). Or wear your shoes loose and untied—even when walking through the airport.

Peter Bakwin, a veteran multiday trail runner, observed a multiday race and offered the following: "I noticed a lot of the multiday runners had the toes cut out of their shoes. We camped next to one runner, and she had several pair like that and her shoes were probably two sizes bigger than you would normally use. She changed her shoes and socks frequently, rotating socks to get dry ones. I also noticed that a lot of the six-day guys were using very thin nylon stockings under their regular socks." Trauma shears make short work of cutting shoes and should be available at any race that has medical support.

Off with the Toes

If you choose to cut the toes out of your shoes, use an EMT scissors or utility shears, not a knife. Plan ahead and have a pair in your medical kit. Using a knife can lead to injury when trying to cut through tough shoe uppers. Here are a few tips:

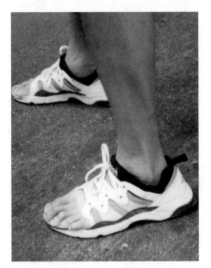

As odd as it may look, cutting the toes off shoes helps prevent common foot problems.

■ Cut from just below the bottom pair of eyelets or the trim piece of fabric that the eyelets go through.

■ Cut down to where the upper joins the sole, from one side around to the other side.

■ Trim as much as necessary to clear the toes.

■ If trimming the heels, keep the top part of the heel counter. Trim under this down to where the upper joins the sole.

■ Use duct tape to cover any rough edges.

Ray Zirblis writes from the experience of 24-hour and multiday stage races. He knows first-hand that foot swelling can trouble racers: "After the Orlander Park 24-Hour, my feet are typically quite swollen for four or five days. Air and auto travel home is always excruciating. Once home, I keep a bucket of ice water by my bed and every couple of hours, when those 'dogs begin to bark,' I get up and soak them. During my first 100-milers, I had a house by a stream and would sleep out by the bank so I could roll over and dunk them periodically."

When I did a 72-hour road race, I learned that a quick 20-minute nap every six hours helped me stay sharp. From 12 hours on, I took these quick "cat naps" for the remaining 60 hours, and during each nap I slightly elevated my feet—with my shoes off.

Going into a multiday event without knowing the best way to care for your feet and how to fix blisters or a turned ankle can spell disaster. Practice before your event and as the preceding chapter suggests, if you have a team or crew, or are on a team or crew, learn everything you can about how to take care of and fix your feet.

Tips for Multiday Events

- Cut the toes out of your shoes (if the location and terrain allow). A piece of Lycra or other stretch material can be glued over the hole to keep out trash.

- Frequently ice your feet or immerse them in ice water during occasional break periods.

- Elevate your feet when resting.

- Rotate your socks to keep your feet as dry as possible.

- Have extra shoes a size or two larger than normal, with interchangeable insoles.

- If you cannot change into larger shoes, start with shoes larger than normal and add a flat insole to help them fit from the start. Remove the insole as your foot swells.

- Use different thicknesses of socks.

- Use anti-inflammatory medications.

- Change shoes and socks frequently.

- Use very thin nylon stockings under regular socks.

- Use Super Salve, Bag Balm, Brave Soldier Antiseptic Healing Ointment, or a similar ointment to keep your feet as healthy as possible.

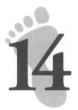

Teamwork & Crew Support

There may be times when you are involved in a team sport or a sport that utilizes a crew. Adventure racing is typically done as a team. Backpacking and hiking, while not team sports per se, may be done as a group. Crew support is found in ultramarathon events, adventure racing, and team sports: football, soccer, and so on. Before your race or activity, develop a plan, draw up a list of supplies, and clarify all the responsibilities of each team or crew member. And be sure to discuss your group's notion of teamwork.

Teamwork

Any time you are with a group, teamwork is vital. You are only as strong as your weakest member and as fast as your slowest member. If you have a crew supporting you and you need foot care, can any crew member manage your feet—or only one? Do team members know how to care for each other's feet as well as their own?

For adventure racing, this is of particular importance. As you train and race, your team will learn from each other's strengths and build on each other's weaknesses. It may sound easy, but this aspect is rated as one of the most complex and difficult of all adventure-racing components. Each team member must have some degree of skill at all of the disci-

176

plines—including foot care. The same can be said for all members of a backpack or hike. The story of one team's experience during an adventure race will illustrate this point.

Patty Hintz, a member of Team R.E.A.R., participated in a two-day adventure race in the Shasta Trinity Alps. She describes the race:

> The mileage for the running section was about 35 miles and one of my teammates had a problem with blisters. Being an experienced ultrarunner I brought along extra Spenco 2nd Skin. When she said blisters, I had no idea we were talking both heels, both forefeet, and multiple toes on each foot! We had three different types of tape to put over the 2nd Skin. I first tried moleskin—but a few miles later it was off. Next was cloth tape, but it did not hold either. Finally, I remembered the duct tape in our team's mandatory gear. I don't know how she managed, but she said her feet felt 100 percent better. She was able to continue the race and the duct tape never came off.

This story is important in that Patty had anticipated foot problems and was prepared. She knew the value of 2nd Skin and knew how to tape the feet. She also knew how to improvise. If she had been on a team where no one knew how to properly drain blisters and tape over them, they may not have finished the two-day event. Patty describes some problems they encountered:

> Later we talked about what caused the blisters. [My teammate] had great running type socks to reduce friction. Her shoes had plenty of break-in time and fit her feet properly. I personally think it was not enough experience with time on her feet. I honestly feel if your shoes fit properly and are the right type of shoe for the way you run, you wear appropriate socks, and spend time breaking in a new pair of shoes before you race in them, blisters are still going to come until your feet have enough distance and time to toughen up. Until then, I'm a firm believer in duct tape and 2nd Skin. As far as my teammate's feet, I'm happy to say they healed very quickly—in about a week.

Planning for Foot Care

People participating in the same activity or on the same team would be wise to sit down before an event, particularly if it is your first or second event together, or your first multiday event, and talk about foot care. Who has the most foot-care experience? What is the best way to prepare your feet—pre-event taping, toughening your skin, better socks, and/or better fitting shoes? As Patty asks, "Does each member have enough time on their feet to toughen them for the distance?" What is the best method to use when fixing blisters? How about really big blisters? What is the minimum amount of foot-care knowledge expected of each person? What foot-care gear will you carry and how much of each item? Foot-care kits are useless if only one person knows how to use the materials in them. Who then will fix that person's feet if problems develop? And who will manage the team's feet if that person is injured or has to be pulled from the race?

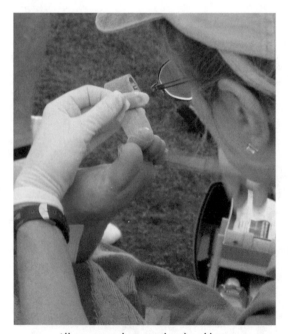

All team members need to be able to work on each other's feet. Here, a teammate wraps Coban over 2nd Skin on a toe blister.

A resource for crews and medical support personnel is the *Foot Care Field Manual,* which will incorporate many of the treatment ideas from this book. Its focus will be on helping crews and medical support teams know what to do to get their athlete back onto the course or into the game. Information on this pocket size manual can be found at **www.fixingyourfeet.com**.

Planning should also include preparing a foot-care kit. The chapter "Foot-Care Kits" (page 312) includes a list of what to include in your kit.

Team Responsibilities

You need to know how to use each item in your foot-care kit. Each member of the team should know how to tape their feet to prevent and fix blisters. Each team member should work at finding what is best for their feet—lubricants or powders, two pairs of socks or one pair, double layer socks or single layer, the best way to lace their shoes for specific foot problems, and finding the best fitting shoes for their feet. It is the responsibility of the whole team to be sure each member is adequately trained in proper foot care. It can mean the difference between a good race and just finishing—or even not finishing.

Crew Support

If you will be participating in an event where you have crew support to help you at aid stations, be sure to discuss foot-care issues with them before the event. Let them know if there will be shoe or sock changes at particular aid stations, and if so, what specific shoes or socks you will want. Let them know all of the following:

- How to take your shoes and socks off to avoid making any foot problems worse
- How to put new shoes and socks back on
- What powders and/or lubricants you use and where on your feet you use them
- How tight you like your shoes tied and whether you use single or double knots
- How you want to deal with hot spots, blisters, toenails, or other unique problems

Practice this with your crew at home, well in advance of the run. By trial and error find what works and what doesn't work. It is important to know the amount of time these activities will take.

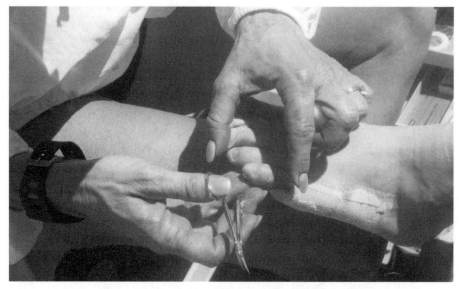

Denise Jones tapes feet at the Western States 100-Mile Endurance Run.

When arriving in the aid station, let them know what you need for your feet. Advise them of any hot spots or blisters. Never let them pull shoes off your feet without proper unlacing. This action, however unintentional, can rupture a blister or cause increased pain to already hurting feet. A shoehorn can be a lifesaver—use it to easily slide the heel out of and into the back of the shoe without too much pressure on sore and tender heels.

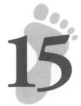

159 Ways to Prevent Blisters

Most athletes hold a common misconception about blisters—that blisters are simply a fact of life that one must learn to live with. Most athletes try tips that they have learned from others. If those don't work, they move on to another idea. Most try for a while, then give up and spend the rest of their life fixing their inevitable blisters. The fact is there are many ways to prevent blisters.

Adventure racer Dan O'Shea spent eight years learning what works for him in preventing blisters: "I have trained my feet for the stress of my sport, and they have a tough outer layer. For races, I use tincture of benzoin, followed by Sports Slick lubricant, and then a double-sock system." At the 1999 Beast of the East Adventure Race he raced with two first-timers whose feet were hardly conditioned to the rigors of a five-day race. After two days of racing Dan found that "both these individuals had blisters on top of blisters and could walk only with great pain." Dan and teammate Harold Zundel, both former navy SEALs and experienced racers, had maybe one blister between the two of them. Over the years he has learned different blister prevention techniques that work best on his feet. But he also realizes that what works for him may change over time as he gets new or different shoes, as his feet change, and as he participates in different types of events under changing conditions. Dan has the right approach—keep on learning and always be open to new blister prevention ideas.

Understand that while the blister prevention techniques you currently use may work today, they may not work tomorrow. I have patched the feet of many ultramarathoners and adventure racers who claim to have never had problems before. Knowing what options are available will help you be prepared. The ideas that follow show the improvising spirit of athletes. They were submitted by athletes, from casual to professional, involved in all types of sports. Try one or two, and then try a few more to find the ones that work for you.

Things You Do to Your Feet

Many athletes believe they that what they do to their feet helps prevent blisters. They have identified many options that are worth trying.

1. I pamper my feet with a pedicure. *Veronica Williams*

2. Give yourself foot massages whenever you can. *Karen Borski*

3. I keep my feet as soft as a baby's bottom. *Dave Scott*

4. Form calluses on your feet.

5. Get rid of calluses.

6. Keep your toenails clipped short. *Pat & Walt Radney*

7. Buff your toenails to get rid of all rough spots.

8. Lightly sandpaper your feet every few days. *Mike Snow*

9. I don't get blisters when my feet are wet! I even dip my feet in streams. *Lisa Demoney*

10. Keep your feet dry by changing socks whenever possible. *Mike Snow*

11. Try to keep your feet dry, air them out at breaks, and change from wet socks to dry ones. *Cynthia Taylor-Miller*

12. Wash your feet every night when out on a hiking trip. *Karen Borski*

13. I learned to wash my feet as seldom as possible and wear the same socks most of the time. My feet developed a protective layer of dead skin and dirt that made them nearly bullet-proof. Blisters and abrasions never developed. *Andrew Perdas*

14. For a week before I pack or race, I soak the soles of my feet in rubbing alcohol. *George Cole*

15. One way to prevent blisters sounds strange but works. Boil oak or hickory bark or twigs in water for 5 to 15 minutes. Allow the water to cool. This makes a mild solution of tannic acid. Soaking feet in this solution will "tan" the skin on your feet and will help prevent blisters. *Carl Schmid*

16. Toughen the skin on your feet by walking and running bare-foot on grass, dirt, and sand. *Matt Mahoney*

17. The more you run the tougher your feet will get. *Mike Snow*

18. Two months before a race, do lots of running sessions with bare feet on sand. *Mike Snow*

19. Blisters and most other foot problems can be avoided alto-gether by hiking in bare feet.

20. My feet may have been in better shape from the running, but they weren't tough enough to deal with the stress that a pack was causing. You must train your feet also. *Brick Robbins*

Things You Apply to Your Feet

There are many things you can apply to your feet to help prevent blisters. Lubricants and tape are two of the most popular. Powders are a distant third. Remember that whatever you apply to your feet will react to what you put around your feet. When you apply a lubricant, your socks will pick up some of it, and more applications will be necessary. Tape works well, but tape applied poorly can be pulled loose as you pull on your socks.

21. Use a callus cream to soften calluses and prevent friction and resulting blisters.

22. Use Bag Balm as a lubricant to reduce friction. *Robert Blackwell*

23. Apply lanolin to your feet.

24. Apply Udder Balm as a lubricant.

25. Use BlisterShield Roll-On as a lubricant.

26. Use BlisterShield Miracle Powder to reduce friction.

27. Apply Gurney Goo as a lubricant.

28. Use BodyGlide lubricant.

29. Use Sports Slick lubricant each time you change your socks. *Dan O'Shea*

30. Apply Vaseline to your feet. *Annie, Phil Mislinski & Bob Slate*

31. Use Avon's Silicone Glove cream to reduce friction.

32. Coat your feet with Hydropel Sports Ointment.

33. Use Chris Koch's Secret Formula of Vaseline, antibacterial ointment, and antifungal cream as a lubricant.

34. We plastered our feet in a substance called Sudocrem twice a day during a big race. Primarily designed to prevent diaper rash, this antiseptic healing cream leaves an oily trace on your feet and lasts for ages. *Brian Elliot*

35. Use foot powder at every opportunity. *Karen Borski*

36. Use Odor-Eater's Foot Powder to absorb moisture.

37. Use Gold Bond Powder—it is an indispensable cure-all for blisters.

38. Use Zeasorb super-absorbent powder on your feet.

39. I use strapping tape.

40. Apply 5-inch strips of "cloth" style duct tape on the heels, the bottom front of the foot, and the right and left toes. *John H*

41. Duct tape known hot spots or problem areas. *George Cole, Bret Edge & Jeffrey Olson*

42. Duct tape really does fix everything. Placed over second skin, or other sterile bandaging, it prevents wear on the skin. *Sandra Kemper*

43. Use Leukotape as a pretape.

44. Use Kineso Tex tape on your feet.

45. Use Bunhead's Gel Toe Caps.

46. Johnson & Johnson Elastikon tape is great preventative medicine! It is porous and easier on your skin than duct tape. *Suzi Cope & Pat Wellington*

47. Apply Johnson & Johnson athletic tape over the spots that have been a problem in the past. *Karl King*

48. Put Band-Aid Blister Relief on any blister-prone spots prior to any race.

49. Apply Band-Aid Blister Relief strips around your toes to prevent toe blisters. *Scott Weber*

50. Use tincture of benzoin to bond Blister Relief pads to your problem spots. *Jeff Wold*

51. Three days before an event, I apply an antiperspirant Ban Roll-on to all skin surfaces up to the ankles, especially between the toes. *George Cole*

52. Put a roll-on or gel antiperspirant on your feet prior to a race and when ever you change socks. *Kier*

53. I use antiperspirant Ban Roll-On every morning of the event before I put on my socks. *George Cole*

54. Spray Mueller's Tuffner Clear Spray on your feet to toughen your skin.

55. Apply Tuf-Foot to toughen and protect your feet.

56. Apply multiple coats of tincture of benzoin to your feet as a skin toughener.

57. Use Tom Crawford's Lipton Tea and Betadine Soak as a skin toughener.

58. Use Andrew Lovy's formula of A and D ointment, Vaseline, Desitin ointment, vitamin E cream, and aloe vera cream.

59. Apply New-Skin Liquid Bandage in several layers over hot spots. *Kojac & Plodder*

60. Used clear nail polish in layers over hot spots. *Kojac*

61. Put moleskin over hot spots.

62. Use Spenco 2nd Skin covered with moleskin.　*Rob Langsdorf*

63. Use adhesive felt. It is thicker than moleskin and sticks better.

64. Put a patch of lamb's wool on a bruised, sore, or blistered area, and secure it to the foot with duct tape.　*Scott Weber*

Things You Put Around Your Feet

What you put around your feet is one of the most important factors in blister prevention. The wrong type of socks, shoes, or boots that fit wrong create pressure points and blisters. Modifying your footwear can help. This is an area where trying different ideas can really pay off.

65. Wear two pair of thin socks.　*Buzz Burrell*

66. Use two types of socks: a thin liner sock made of silk or polypropylene with your favorite outer sock on top.　*Dan O'Shea*

67. Wear three pairs of socks: the first pair is a wicking sock, then the others are regular socks.　*Matthew Jankowicz*

68. Use two CoolMax socks that allow motion between the two layers and not with the feet.　*Paul Alsop*

69. Wear nylons under wool socks for hiking.　*Mary Gorski*

70. Wear rock climber's socks. They are thin and fit snugly.　*Will Uher*

71. Always wear SmartWool ultra-thin running socks—they are great at wicking, dry quickly, and cause no irritation.　*Phil Mislinski*

72. Wear liner socks.

73. Use one of the new socks with an antiblister system.

74. Wear Gore-Tex fabric socks.

75. Avoid cotton socks—they retain moisture.

76. Wear socks with Blister-Guard's Teflon fibers.

77. Wear SealSkinz WaterBlocker socks.

78. Wear Injinji toe socks.

79. Wear polyester dress socks, the slicker the better.

80. Don't wear polypropylene sock liners. Until I threw mine away, I had horrible blisters which I had to duct tape. *BettySue Allen*

81. CoolMax socks do an excellent job of wicking moisture away from the feet. *Paul Alsop*

82. Wear socks inside out. The seam that goes across the toes can rub the tops and sides of the toes and cause blisters. *Cynthia Taylor-Miller*

83. Duct tape your socks in areas where you tend to blister. *Rick Lewis*

84. The heel is the first part of the sock to wear thin. Get new socks before they get too threadbare. *Kevin Corcoran*

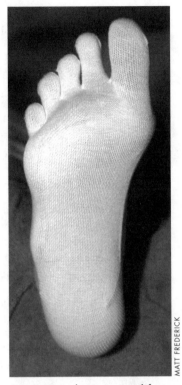

Injinji toe sock over a taped foot.

85. I've had good luck putting pieces of lamb's wool coated with lanolin between the toes. This soft, fibrous padding is usually available in the foot section of most drugstores and pharmacies. The natural lanolin in the wool was a breakthrough, because no matter how well or completely I tape my toes, I blistered between them. *Ray Zirblis*

86. To prevent heel blisters at the bottom back edge of the heel, where the insole meets the foot, put a small piece of lamb's wool or sheepskin on the edge of the insole to fill that space. In a pinch you can cut the top off rag socks or by unraveling the sock and getting a bunch of yarn—just use the whole wad. *Joanne Lennox*

87. Weave strips of lamb's wool between your toes and around the tips of your toes, and add more as needed. Wash it occasionally to restore its loft and cushioning. *Michael Henderson*

88. Check a new pair of shoes or boots for problem areas, even if they are the same brand and size as your last pair. *Joanne Lennox*

89. Be sure to smooth the heels of your socks, and check the heels of your insoles and the inside of your heel counters for folds and worn or torn material. *Jay Hodde*

90. Duct tape rough areas inside your boots.

91. Use ENGO Performance Patches on potential problem areas of your insoles and shoes.

92. Use well-cushioned shoes. *Veronica Williams*

93. Above all else, make sure the shoes fit. *Buzz Burrell*

94. Get boots that fit properly. *Cynthia Taylor-Miller*

95. To keep your feet dry, look for shoes and boots with good ventilation. *Cynthia Taylor-Miller*

96. Unless it's quite cold I wear well-ventilated trail running shoes when on the trail. *George Cole*

97. Once I find a pair of shoes that fits well and works for my running style and choice of terrain, I buy at least six pair. *Phil Mislinski*

98. If you haven't worn your old boots for sometime, always take at least one walk in them before going on a major hike. Your foot may have changed and it may need to get reacquainted with the boot before making a long hike with it. *Rob Langsdorf*

99. Switch from leather boots to running shoes for hiking and modify them with your knife if they feel too tight or hurt. *Kojac*

100. Replace worn-out shoes. *Kojac*

101. Use shoes that are tested for the event and the distance. Have one model for cold weather and another for trails in warm and/or wet conditions. *Doug McKeever*

102. For hiking I use an old pair of combat boots with the toes cut off about 3 inches across the top of the toes. Have a shoe shop sew a strip of leather about 1 inch wide across the boot to reinforce the opening. This makes all five toes visible on both feet and saves the toes. *Billie M. Thrash*

103. Once I switched to another pair of shoes the blisters went away. Many shoes breathe better than others and are better on your feet.

104. To drain out sweat and water, use a red hot nail to burn drain holes on the sides of your shoes right at the sock liner height where the shoe bends. *Jim Stroup*

105. Use Superfeet insoles. *Walt & Pat*

106. Well-made orthotics will help prevent blisters.

107. Wear shoe gaiters to keep rocks, dust, and dirt out of the shoes, which means that the socks stay cleaner longer. *Paul Alsop*

108. Change to stretchy shoelaces to eliminate hot spots on top of your feet.

Things You Do in Combination

Some blister prevention ideas work best in combination with other ideas: Vaseline and wicking socks, tincture of benzoin to hold tape on the feet, skin tougheners and double-layer socks. The list goes on and on, everything from using an antiperspirant to using motor oil!

109. Keep your feet soft and supple. I get a pedicure at least once a month to smooth out all calluses and rough spots, and put creams on my feet on a daily basis. When I hit the trails or roads, I use foot powder. Things have improved greatly. *Dave Littlehales*

110. Vaseline your feet, and then pull on ankle length nylons, followed by socks and then shoes. *Geraldine Wales*

111. First, duct tape all problem areas, and then apply a light coating of lubricant to your feet, put the first sock on each foot, apply more lubricant to the foot section of the socks, and put on the second pair of socks. *Dalton Pulsipher Jr.*

112. Use Ultimax socks and a thin coat of Vaseline. *Jim Stroup*

113. Apply medicated A and D ointment to your feet the night before a race, and then the socks you will run in the next day. Reapply the ointment in the morning and use the same socks. *Scott Snyder*

114. Wear shoes that fit a little big and wear double-layer socks. And stay well hydrated. *Jay Hodde*

115. Apply tincture of benzoin to the bottom and sides of the foot. Then with the foot in a relaxed position, layer strips of athletic tape from the back of the heel to the front of the foot, with each piece slightly overlapping the previous piece. *Charles Steele*

116. Spray your feet with Cramer's Tuf Skin, followed by Hydropel Silicone Protective Ointment. *Dr. Billy Tolan*

117. Use a combination of thin CoolMax socks, frequent sock changes, relubricating with Bag Balm every 25 miles, and continuous fluid and salt intake. *Bill Ramsey*

118. Spray your feet with New-Skin Liquid Bandage, and wear nylon hose and then double-layer socks, all this inside of extra-long and extra-wide shoes. *Nikki Robinson*

119. Spray the soles of your feet with Cramer's Tuf-Skin or an equivalent. Two coats are better. Let each coat dry a minute or so until tacky, then roll on a pair of the two-layer CoolMax double-layer socks. The tacky spray causes the inner layer of the two-layer sock to bond to your foot. All the slippage, and friction, thus occurs between the two layers of the sock, or between the sock and the shoe. *Pierre Redmond*

120. Clean your feet thoroughly. Coat your heels, toes, and soles with tincture of benzoin. After it dries, apply a layer of Avon Silicone Glove, followed by double-layer socks. Reapply every four to six hours and change socks at the same time. *Marvin Skagerberg*

121. Wear good shoes and socks that fit properly. *Dennis Halpin*

122. Wear Duraspun acrylic socks with lots of foot powder.

123. Use duct tape, foot powder, and synthetic socks. *David Burroughs*

124. Wear CoolMax socks, with duct tape on the sock over the areas where the hot spots are or will be, and a second pair of socks over this combination. You must remove the duct tape from the sock and soak the sock in hot soapy water as soon as possible to remove the duct tape glue. *Rick*

125. I pretape my feet in areas where I know from past experience I have had blisters and use shoes that on nontaped feet have not caused blisters on shorter runs. It isn't taping or the shoes—it's both. *Doug McKeever*

126. Shave the hair off your feet and duct-tape them before you leave the house.

127. I recommend new motor oil, basic cheap oil works great. No special weight, but I try to stay away from oils with additives. Then cheap men's 50/50 cotton-polyester socks from any discount department store. The 100 percent synthetic seem to work also, but I'm too cheap to buy them. Remember though, the oil must be new since used oil is a carcinogenic. *Ray Krolewicz*

128. The night before a run apply Cramer Tuf-Skin. In the morning rub on Vaseline and coat with baby powder, followed by nylon socks, more powder, and then thick socks. *Scott Rafferty*

129. Dry feet and good clean socks are the best prevention for blisters.

130. I first spray the bottom, sides, and blister-prone parts of my feet with tincture of benzoin and let it dry. At first I used to cut strips of duct tape but now use 3M Microfoam tape. Stretch it slightly as you put it on and smooth out any bumps. *G. Velasco*

131. I use women's nylon ankle stockings on my feet first, followed by double- or single-layer CoolMax socks. *Ray Zirblis*

132. I wear a CoolMax liner sock with either Thorlo CoolMax blend light hiking socks summer or SmartWool hiking socks winter. *George Cole*

133. Change the liner and sock for a second pair about once every two hours or less if it's really warm and let the original pair dry out. *George Cole*

134. Wash off your feet at night and coat with Vaseline. *Walt & Pat*

Things You Do in General

In addition to doing things to your feet, applying things to your feet, being careful to what you put around your feet, and there are other ideas that are helpful in preventing blisters. The ideas here run the gamut from lacing techniques, hydration, proper shoe and boot fit, and regular changes of socks.

135. Drink a lot of water to stay hydrated. *John H*

136. Stay properly hydrated with electrolytes to maintain good sodium levels. *Karl King*

137. Learn different lacing techniques to prevent your feet from slipping inside the shoes.

138. Relace your shoelaces in a different lace configuration to take the pressure off a hot spot. *Pat & Walt Radney*

139. The key is prevention, think of boot, socks, epidermis, and lower skin layers as a "system" and treat the whole system. *Tom McGinnis*

140. Elevate your feet at breaks and at night to keep swelling down.

141. Run without socks to keep your feet from sliding around in your shoes and get a better grip on the soles of your shoes. *Matt Mahoney*

142. Stop and check out "hot spots" before they turn into blisters. *Rob Langsdorf*

143. Slow down if you feet start to overheat. Often this allows the feet to cool enough to keep from blistering. *Rob Langsdorf*

144. If you are hiking in wet boots and socks, slow your pace a bit to reduce pressure on the skin of your feet. *Karen Borski*

145. Rotate between several pairs of shoes. *Jon Drury*

146. For extreme heat, I cut up a space blanket on all the nonwhite parts of my shoes and under the insole to reduce the heat that causes blisters. *Clive Saffery*

147. I wore boots that were slightly too large so that during the course of a hike, as my feet naturally swelled, they wouldn't become too tight and rub.

148. I started hiking with a pack on every weekend. After initial blisters, calluses finally developed, which helped toughen my feet.

149. Don't sleep in damp socks. *Karen Borski*

150. Don't hike ultra-long days in wet boots. *Karen Borski*

151. Wet feet are less a problem than is the dust, dirt, and tiny pebbles that work their way through your shoes. The mesh upper allows the grit in, and the sweat from your feet turns it to a mucky ooze that just invites trouble. Take a break at the aid stations and remove your shoes and socks, wipe your feet, pound out the dirt in the socks, and put everything back on. *Jay Hodde*

152. Allow your feet dry out as often as possible, including taking shoes-off breaks when out for a long hike. *Karen Borski*

153. Take your boots and socks off once an hour, religiously, to air your feet. *Jeffrey Olson*

154. If blisters persist, get new shoes. *Karen Borski*

155. I trace the outline of my feet on an 8-by-11-inch paper after doing a 100-miler and sketch in the blisters, noting any antiblister techniques I used. This helps me remember what I've tried and what worked or didn't. *Ray Zirblis*

156. The guy at the outfitters who helped me fit my boots correctly saved my feet.

157. Go for long hikes with your feet soaking wet. The idea is to get blisters started, let them heal, and do it again. *Bruce*

158. The best way I've found to prevent blisters is to get blisters. I don't do anything to avoid blisters on training runs and actually welcome it when I do get a blister because I know my feet are getting tougher. On race day it's different—then I go for the double socks, gaiters, comfortable shoes, etc. *Scott Diamond*

And finally, ending on a humorous note, one more way to prevent blisters.

159. I have discovered a 100-percent foolproof way of avoiding blisters. Its beauty lies in its simplicity, its effectiveness is unparalleled by any remedy to which I've been exposed, and it works just as well in the marathon/ultramarathon world as it does in adventure racing. Here it is: At the start of the race, as everyone takes off, you elevate both feet on a log, an ottoman, a slavish support crew member, or whatever and if you can stay there until the race is over, blisters are guaranteed not to get you. *David Schmitt*

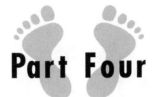

Part Four

Treatments

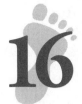

16

Treating Your Feet

The 4th Law of Running Injuries:
Virtually all running injuries are curable.
Only a minute fraction of true running injuries are not entirely
curable by quite simple techniques.
—Tim Noakes, MD, *The Lore of Running*[18]

No matter how hard we try to prevent problems with our feet, there may come a time when they need repairing. Then you become reactive. The following chapters explain how to fix typical foot problems. It is always best to know how to fix problems before they develop. Beginning a long trail run or a multiday hike without preparing for the possibility of blisters, a sprained ankle, or other potential injury is foolhardy. One or two unexpected blisters at the wrong time can spell the end to a long-anticipated event.

In 2000, I conducted a survey of runners, ultrarunners, triathletes, hikers, and adventure racers. While not a formal scientific survey, the 214 responses showed some interesting results:

- Athlete's foot is more common in males.
- Black toenails affect 71 percent.

- Calluses affect 49 percent.

- Ingrown toenails have affected 32 percent.

- Morton's foot affects 30 percent.

- Sprained ankles affect 11 percent now and have affected 36 percent in the past. Many participants have experienced this more than 15 times—the highest was 30 times!

- Missing toenails have affected 57 percent.

- Achilles tendinitis affects 11 percent now and has affected 25 percent in the past.

- Plantar fasciitis affects 17 percent now and has affected 30 percent in the past.

- Orthotics are worn by 36 percent.

As you can see from the results, most of us are not immune to injuries or problems with our feet. Of particular interest was that many of those surveyed had more two or more problems with their feet at the same time. What the survey told me was that athletes need to know how to treat common foot ailments—not just what they now have, but what they might experience as a result of their activity.

The Marathon des Sables, an extreme six-day, self-supported race in the Moroccan desert, treats runners to 150 miles of sand, sand, and more sand; 200-foot sand dunes; rocky roads with small odd-shaped stones; heat that sucks the moisture out of skin; and winds and sandstorms that torment every inch of your being. Robert Nagle, a highly experienced EcoChallenge adventure racer, ran the race in 1997 and had only one blister. He commented that "many of the participants have neither the experience nor knowledge of foot care for ultras—so they suffer mightily." The name of the game is to plan ahead to finish well and with healthy feet. If you don't, you are at a disadvantage right from the start.

In 1996, Dave Covey, an experienced ultrarunner, participated in a competitive and challenging 25-day 600k wilderness trek across Western Australia that stressed his feet beyond his wildest imagination. While working in a walking and backpacking shoe store, he studied the different types of boots and selected a nylon-and-leather boot with a Gore-Tex fabric interior. The combination of high temperatures, long pants, and wearing heavy-duty nylon gaiters to protect his legs from the spiny vegetation made his legs sweat constantly. With his feet always wet, and the terrain very uneven and rocky, his feet were subject to extreme punishment. Changing into dry wicking–style socks every two hours helped for the first two days. By the third day blisters had developed on the bottoms of his toes. Moleskin simply would not adhere to the wet skin. By the end of the eighth day he rested his feet for a few days to try to dry out the blisters. He then used Betadine and duct tape on the toes. By the eighteenth day, the skin finally began to callous over and during the last six days of the trek, he did not have to use any tape. Dave gave his boots high marks for comfort, realizing the blisters were caused by other factors.

In the above two cases, Robert and Dave had done their homework. They knew what their feet needed to complete their extreme event. They planned and were prepared. Whether we are doing something similar or something much, much easier, we too need to have a basic understanding of treatments to fix out feet.

Some things are very basic. When your feet are tired, you have several ways to help them feel better. When changing socks, stopping for lunch, or whenever possible, take a few minutes and massage your feet and check for any hot spots. A short soak in an icy stream or in a bucket of cold water can revitalize tired feet. When you sit down to change socks or shoes after being on your feet for any great length of time, elevating your feet above the level of your heart will help reduce swelling of the feet. While hiking or on adventure races, try to wash your feet with soap and water at least once per day, preferably in the evening.

Other things are more detailed and complex and are included in the chapters that follow. The information includes descriptions of problems, ways to treat them, products that can help relieve or solve them, and, in some cases, exercises to strengthen the affected areas. Read the chapters that pertain to your injury history, and try the treatments and products to find those that will resolve your problems.

Blisters

Blisters start out as hot spots. If caught in time and treated, hot spots can be controlled. Left to their own, they will develop into an irritating blister that can stop you in your tracks, end your athletic event, and sideline you for weeks. Hot spots are simple to prevent and treat. Blisters are different. Many athletes think there is one way to patch blisters. This chapter will show you many different ways to manage pesky blisters. Some are simple and quick. Others are complex and take more time—because they are meant to last during an ultramarathon or adventure race.

Part of caring for blisters is to also identify and eliminate the problem that caused them in the first place. One runner reported having developed the first blisters he had ever gotten while running, though he didn't notice them until afterwards. After a 50-mile trial run he had two identical blisters, one on the tip of each little toe. Here is where detective work can get tricky. The blisters could have been caused by the seam welt over the little toes on the inside of the sock (a very common problem in a very common spot). It could have been the fit of the shoes—perhaps the shoes and/or the toe box were too short. The toenails could have been the culprits if they were too long, catching on the socks, and making them bunch up at that point. Or the downhills could have been the culprit. Then too, the runner could have had a problem with his little toes—perhaps they were longer than normal or angled in such a way to be more prone to friction. Be aware of all the factors that go into the fit of your shoes and socks and how everything on and around your feet works as a unit. Simply patching a blister and continuing on is fixing only part of the problem.

Treating blisters takes time and practice. Denise Jones tells of a runner at the Death Valley Badwater Ultramarathon:

> He had a combination of the wrong socks (all cotton), shoes that became too small once his feet swelled after 115 miles, and virtually no adequate tape with which to repair his throbbing feet. After nearly an hour and a half, I was able to drain and dress his blisters and cut the toes out of his shoes so that the swollen nubs—his toes—could become less crowded. I was pleased to learn that after that session of repair, he was able to complete the distance and finish the race. He thanked me over and over for helping him.

Hot Spots

Most runners experience hot spots in the areas where they are susceptible to blisters forming. The area will become sore and red—thus, the name "hot spot." You may also experience a stinging or burning sensation. Around the reddened area will be a paler area that enlarges inward to where the skin is being rubbed.[19] The area becomes elevated because the surface skin is lifted as it fills with fluid. The hot spot has then become a blister.

When you feel a hot spot develop, check your socks to be sure they have not bunched up, retie your laces, and check inside your shoe to be sure there is no debris that could be an irritant.

Treating Hot Spots

You must deal with these hot spots before they become blisters. By the time the hot spot has developed enough to be felt, protection is necessary. Take the time to deal with hot spots as you feel them develop. Continuing to run or hike on them will only make them worse. Untreated hot spots usually turn into blisters, which are harder to treat. Use your choice of one of the tapes or blister care products described in this book to protect the area. If you have used lubricants or powders on your feet, clean the affected area with an alcohol wipe before applying tape, adhesive felt, or moleskin.

Hot spots typically develop from pressure caused by your footwear or socks. Examine your shoes or boots to determine whether you can modify them to remove the pressure point causing the problem. You may have to make a slit or cut out a small section in the side or toe of the shoe. Start with a small cut or hole and enlarge it as necessary. Be sure your socks are not bunched up and creating pressure points. Run your hands inside the socks to remove any loose lint balls. After putting on your socks, use your hands to smooth the material around the shape of each foot.

Beyond Hot Spots: Blisters

Basically, blisters are an injury. And as we all know, blisters can be painful. One blister in a sensitive place on the foot can easily ruin an otherwise good day. Blisters have often destroyed months of training and hundreds of dollars spent on a major event. Several blisters can drain your energy and reduce a runner to a walker or a hiker to a plodder, which in turn tends to create more blisters, which then slows forward motion even more. Too many athletes fail to educate themselves about blister prevention and how to do adequate blister care. Many runners and hikers think blisters are

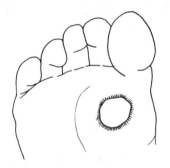

unavoidable and simply a part of the running or hiking process. Sometimes I think we should offer an award to the folks with the biggest blisters! Yet, somehow, when I remove a runner's shoe at the Highway 49 aid station at Western States and the skin falls off half of each foot, I realize the runner should not get an award, but an education on good foot care.

An Experiment of One

Ultrarunner Mark Williams has learned that the blister issue is an individual one: "What works for one may not work for the other. You must experiment, experiment, and experiment. If something doesn't work, don't try to make it work. I've had some nasty blister issues. I tried taping, Bag Balm, Runner's Lube, and Vaseline, wider shoes, and longer shoes. I think the blister issue is an individual one." Consider a few of the following experiences of a few runners:

- "I get a lot of blisters on my right foot and very few on the left."
- "I constantly get blisters when I run any longer distances of 25-plus miles and only on the side of the two toes next to the big toe on my left foot."
- "Wearing orthotics, I am prone to continual blisters on the inside of my right heal where the foot hits the orthotic."
- "The only blisters I get are on my little or big toes, and then only during races."
- "I never had a blister until today."

Some athletes claim to have feet with skin as soft as a baby's bottom while others take pride in having thick calluses on the bottom of their feet. Both may claim to never blister and yet on another day, in a different race or activity with different conditions and variables, both may blister. Kevin Setnes keeps telling us, "We are each an experiment of one." We need to remember that our feet change. Other blister-causing factors also change race to race—weather conditions, a lack of foot conditioning through training, the body's hydration level, the length of the race, running biomechanics as the runner reacts to a sore hamstring or tight quads, for example, all contribute to potential problems.

Blisters come in a variety of sizes. They start small, from a hot spot, and can continue to grow until they are treated. One blister may not seem like much, but suddenly you have two, and then, maybe three. Multiply the pain of one well-placed blister times three or four, like some people get, and you can imagine how severe a seemingly minor problem can become.

When ultrarunner A. J. Howie did the 1992 Trans-America, he described his blisters as "pepperoni pizza blisters," large enough to make the *Guinness Book of World Records*. Blisters can also become major nightmares. John Supler, participating in the Marathon des Sables, reported, "When I came in my feet were shredded like noodles. And when I woke up, my foot was stuck to my silk sheet, with a pool of yellow pus underneath it, leaking out."

The time and conditions required for blisters to develop will vary from individual to individual. Runners and hikers tend to get either "downhill" blisters on the toes and forefoot caused by friction while going downhill, or "uphill" blisters on the heels and over the Achilles tendons caused by friction while going uphill. Blisters on the heel can also mean the heel cup is too wide. Blisters on the top or front of the toes or the outsides of the outer toes can indicate friction in the toe box.

In 15 years Kevin O'Neall has done 30 marathons and over a dozen ultras. He shares his tries at preventing blisters:

> I have never done a long race without getting blisters. I've tried it all: lubricants, double-layer socks, size D, E, 2E, and 4E New Balance shoes, sandals, and military boots. I use a Dremel drill to sand calluses once or twice weekly, and a hacksaw and grinder to trim the soles near blister zones. I cut into my shoes for extra toe room, and then patch the hole with tape to keep dirt out. I've experimented with every kind of tape there is and used seven different brands of duct tape. Nothing works perfectly.
>
> So what's the miracle? While surfing the Badwater Website, I saw a mention of a toe product used by dancers. Bunheads (**www.bunheads.com**) makes flexible fabric toe socks with a gel lining. Sounds dumb, but I ordered some. The box has a photo of a dainty dancer's leg standing on its toes. So far I've got about 40 miles on one tube with no breakdown. The box says they're washable, but I've run without washing them to see how they'd stand up to sweat and grime.

Kevin attempted the Leadville 100 in 2002 and got hot spots on his right big toe even though I'd applied Elastikon. He rolled a piece of Bunhead Big Tips over the Elastikon and was able to continue until a fall strained a calf muscle and forced him to walk. He eventually missed a cutoff and was out of the run, but the Bunheads kept him in the race up to that point.

The bottom line is that finding what prevents blisters on your feet can take much time and experimentation. It may involve one or more of the prevention measures in the previous chapters. It may also involve using one of the treatments in this chapter.

Blisters 101

A basic understanding of how blisters are formed is necessary to successfully treat them. Heat, friction, and moisture contribute to the formation of blisters. Studies have shown that the foot inside the shoe or boot is exposed to friction at many sites as it experiences motion from side to side, front to back, and up and down. These friction sites also change during the activity as the exercise intensity, movement of the sock, and flexibility of the shoe or boot changes.[20]

The outer epidermis layer of skin receives friction that causes it to rub against the inner dermis layer of skin. This friction between the layers of skin causes a blister to develop. As the outer layer of the epidermis is loosened from the deeper layers, the sac in between becomes filled with lymph fluid. A blister has then developed. If the blister is deep or traumatically stressed by continued running or hiking, the lymph fluid may contain blood. When the lymph fluid lifts the outer layer of epidermis, oxygen and nutrition to this layer is cut off and it becomes dead skin. This outer layer is easily burst. The fluid then drains and the skin loses its natural protective barrier. The underlying skin is raw and sensitive. At this point, the blister is most susceptible to infection.

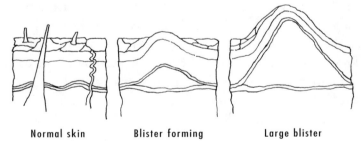

Normal skin   Blister forming   Large blister

The friction against whatever is touching the skin causes the friction between the layers of skin. As identified earlier, the majority of foot problems can be traced back to socks, powders, and lubricants—or the lack of them. In order to prevent blisters, friction must be reduced. Friction can be reduced in three main ways: wearing double-layer socks or one inner and one outer sock, keeping the feet dry by using powders, or using a lubricant to reduce chafing. It has been found that rubbing moist skin tends to produce higher friction than does rubbing skin that is either very dry or very wet.[21] Since the skin blisters more easily when soft and moist, it is important to understand the value of moisture-wicking socks coupled with knowing whether powders and/or lubricants are best for your feet and how to use them. Eliminating pressure points caused by poor-fitting insoles and/or ill-fitting shoes can also reduce friction.

Since your footwear causes blisters, the healing process truly begins when these are removed. If you have the option of a day's layover in camp without shoes and socks, this can speed the healing process and get you back on your feet faster and feeling better. Wearing sandals without socks exposes the blister to the air, which aids in healing.

Try to avoid getting blisters on top of existing blisters. When your skin is healing, protect or cushion the tender area.

Blisters Yesterday, Today & Tomorrow

Most of us face it at one time or another: what worked for us in the past is no longer working. Ultrarunner Marv Skagerberg candidly warns, "Caveat pedis, or let the toes beware. I have completely solved the blister problem 12 times by perfecting various methods that allow me to run for 24 hours and up, blister free. However, the next time out with the exact same method, I have plenty of blisters." He has found that a combination of tincture of benzoin and silicone cream is by far the best for his feet (see the section "Extreme Blister Prevention and Care" (page 220) for his method). Yesterday's method may have worked for years. Today's method may work for years. But then again, as Marv warns, it may not.

"I *personal experience*

had hoped that 15 years as a long-distance runner and backpacker had eliminated the element of surprise in regard to foot problems and their treatment. I was wrong.

"The first day of my 17-day hike required an additional 11-mile climb to the trailhead atop Mt. Whitney's 14,500-foot summit. On the way up, both heels started to blister. A little early in the trip I thought, but not unexpected. I immediately applied my favorite remedy, 2nd Skin. This was to become a daily ritual. The 2nd Skin would ease the soreness and keep the wounds reasonably clean, but the Adhesive Knit that held it in place could not withstand the rigors of such a brutal, rocky trail, and the blisters worsened to over an inch in diameter. Every step was painful, distracting me from the trail's beautiful surroundings. Soon, I ran out of Adhesive Knit and resorted to that trusty standby, duct tape. This kept the dressings in place longer, but after clambering up and over yet another 12,000-foot pass, it too would slip. Then I got a rash from the tape's adhesive and smaller blisters from the tape's edges.

"At my resupply point, nine days into the trip, I stocked up on 2nd Skin and duct tape, and padded the heel cups of my two-year-old 'broken-in' boots with moleskin and more duct tape. This stopped any future heel blistering but pushed my toes forward in the boots just enough to cause a whole new set of foot problems for the final leg of my trip. Some days it just isn't worth getting out of bed!"

**—Tony Burke recalling the way he approached
his 1996 backpack of the 211-mile
John Muir Trail in California's Sierra Nevada**

The late ultrarunner Dick Collins used to have problems with blisters. After trying recommendations from others, including tape, he formed his own conclusion. Dick learned that "anything other than socks on my feet will over time become an irritant." He used only Vaseline on his feet and wore synthetic socks. Having completed 1,037 races, including 238 ultras, he found what worked for him and stuck to it. Like Dick, we each need to learn what works for us and be open to trying new ideas and products that could help keep our feet healthy.

We have no guarantee that what works one day will work another day. Ultrarunner Damon Lease experienced this frustration. By mile 20 of a 50-mile race he was feeling hot spots on his toes. By mile 38 he was reduced to a painful walking state. At the 42.2-mile aid station he made the difficult decision to stop. Damon noted that he "did nothing different in this race than any other ultra." He had used the same shoe and sock combination in other ultras, but this course was steeper with "more loose rocks and rough footing than the others." It happens. The trick is to play with all the variables in training to find what works best for your feet. Then be prepared with additional options in your gear bag.

General Blister Care

From the perspective of runners and hikers, the goal of blister treatments is to make the foot comfortable since often running or hiking must continue. Bryan P. Bergeron, MD, identifies four therapeutic goals of blister management[22]:

He recommends all blister treatments be considered with these four goals in mind.

- avoiding infection
- minimizing pain and discomfort
- stopping further blister enlargement
- maximizing recovery

Ultrarunner Gillian Robinson has learned to "try to pay a lot of attention to healing, so I don't run on wounded feet. Even the worst blisters heals in about five days if you use Neosporin and cover it during the day and leave it uncovered to breathe at night (if it's not too gross). My feet seem to toughen up after blister trauma, so I trim off the dead skin and keep going."

For years, normal blister care has been gauze, moleskin, and Vaseline. Anyone can slap on a piece of moleskin and slather on some Vaseline and hope for the best. But to really fix a blister so you can continue running or hiking is an art. Observing the podiatrists at the finish line of a marathon or ultra, one finds most blister care practices incorporate these three materials.

The time-honored method of blister care uses moleskin to protect the blister. If the blister is intact, cut a piece of moleskin about ½ inch to ¾ inch larger around than the blister with a hole slightly larger than the blister in the center. Press it on the skin around the blister and put an antibiotic ointment, Bag Balm, or medicated Vaseline in the hole over the blister. The final step is to tape a piece of gauze over the moleskin. Adding a piece of adhesive knit or tape over the gauze will help hold it in place.

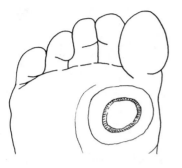

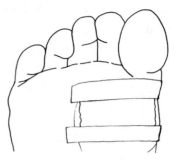

Moleskin with center hole cut out for blister.   Gauze taped over moleskin to protect blister.

Alternatives to moleskin are adhesive felt, one of the tapes identified below, or Spenco Pressure Pads. You can also use one of the tapes or Spenco Skin Knit in place of the gauze. When using tape or moleskin over a blister, apply it as smoothly as possible. Use finger pressure to smooth it evenly across the blister, and then repeat the smoothing process several more times after the initial application. Remember to cut the tape or moleskin large enough to extend well beyond the edges of the blister. The most common failure in using tape or moleskin is not allowing enough necessary for good adherence. The larger the blister, the more the tape or moleskin should extend past its edges.

When using moleskin over blisters, Bill Trolan, MD, recommends using a razor to shave the moleskin, after it is applied, to remove its tiny fibers. The fibers can later catch on socks and pull against the blister.

Basic Blister Repair

If the above treatment does not help or if you must continue running or hiking, take time to repair a blister before it enlarges and ruptures. Dr. Bergeron recommends draining the blister prior to applying a dressing when it is in a weight-bearing area and larger than ⁴⁄₅ inch in diameter.[23] There are two basic ways to drain a blister, one using a needle and the other using a small, sharp scissors or nail clippers.

To drain a blister using the needle method, do the following:

1. Use an alcohol wipe or hydrogen peroxide to clean the skin around the blister.

2. Sterilize a pin or needle with a flame by heating with a match (avoid soot on the tip). Use it to lance two to four puncture holes in a row in the blister. Making a single large hole increases the possibility of the blister roof shearing off as you continue running or hiking.

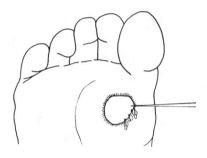

Use a sterilized needle to make several small holes on the outside edges of the blister.

3. Make the puncture holes on the side of the blister where ongoing foot pressure will push out additional fluid, generally to the back of the foot and towards the outside.

4. Use pressure from your fingers to push out the fluid.

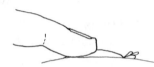

Gently push out the lymph fluid.

5. Blot the fluid away with a tissue.

6. Clean and dry the skin before doing further blister care. The outer layer of dead skin should not be removed.

It is important that the blister not be allowed to refill with fluid. Use one of the blister-care products in the next section to protect the blister. Occasionally recheck the blister and drain it if it has refilled with fluid.

If you are prone to hot spots and blisters, try dabbing on a bit of Anbesol or Kankaid on before patching. These products, sold in drugstores, are numbing medicine for your gums and will also work to numb the painful spots on your feet.

A better method for draining blisters is to use standard nail clippers or small pointed scissors and clip a hole at the edge at the most dependent spot and also at 180 degrees from there. This lets both gravity and capillary action, along with muscular movement, fully empty the blister. The clippers make a V notch, rather than a simple hole. Podiatrist Dan Simpson reports,

"I have never had a complication from this method and the clippers are easier to manipulate than scissors due to the shorter distance from your hand to the business end. The clipper also functions as a built-in depth gauge, preventing too deep an incision."

Another method helps blisters drain better when further hiking or running is required. Ray Zirblis picked up this tip while running the six-day Marathon des Sables in Morocco, and it would be appropriate for stage races or multidays where a runner will need to keep running. Tom Ripley taught him how to do it. At the end of the day's run or other effort, if you find blisters, drain them and add another step: Sterilize a needle and a few inches of thread with alcohol. Then thread the needle and run it and the thread through one side of the blister and out the other, leaving the thread in place with a ¼- to ½-inch tail hanging on either end. The thread acts as a wick to further drain any moisture in the blister while one is running or sleeping. Ray reports, "I found that my blisters dried more thoroughly overnight than normal for me, and the inside was much less raw and less sensitive than usual."

In some cases, you should not attempt to drain blisters. *Do not drain a blister when it is blood-filled.* Doing so creates the risk of a serious infection as bacteria is easily introduced into the dermis layer of skin and into the blood system. Pad around the blister with moleskin or adhesive felt.

Do not drain the blister if the fluid inside appears to be either cloudy or hazy. Normal blister fluid is clear and the change indicates that an infection has set in. If clear, the fluid needs to be drained, an antibiotic ointment applied, and a protective covering applied. Recheck the blister three times a day for signs of the infection returning. Each time you check, apply a new coating of antibiotic ointment and change the dressing. Early treatment can keep the infection from becoming more serious.

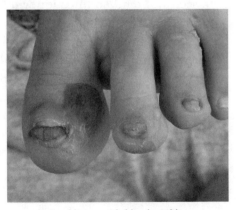

Toe blister with blood visible.
Do not lance blood-filled blisters.

If the blister has ruptured, the degree of repair depends on the condition of the blister's outer covering. Clean around the blister as described below and apply one of the blister-care methods described in the next section. You can treat a ruptured blister—if the skin is generally intact.

If the outer layer of skin is torn off or only a flap of skin is left, carefully cut off the loose skin, clean the area, and cover the new skin with one of the blister-care methods described in the next section. Valerie Doyle uses a hair dryer on the blister when the outer layer of skin has been removed or torn off. She has found the low heat and drying action speeds the healing process.

Preventing Infection

For open blisters, using soap and water, and an antibiotic ointment, Betadine, or hydrogen peroxide is important for avoiding infection. Though you may not use these on an open blister during a run or in the middle of the day while backpacking, at the end of the event or day, take the necessary time to properly treat the open skin. Check your local drugstore for a broad-spectrum antibiotic ointment like Neosporin or Polysporin that provides protection against both gram-positive and gram-negative pathogens. Brave Soldier Wound Healing Ointment is an excellent all-purpose salve to have on hand for blister care.

Recheck blisters daily for signs of infection. An infected blister may be both seen and felt. An infection will be indicated by any of the following: redness, swelling, red streaks up the limb, pain, fever, and pus. Treat the blister as a wound. Clean it frequently and apply an antibiotic ointment. Frequent warm water or Epsom salt soaks can also help the healing process. Stay off the foot as much as possible and elevate it above the level of your heart. If the infection does not seem to subside over 24 to 48 hours, see a doctor.

BLISTER-CARE PRODUCTS

ADHESIVE FELT is available in rolls in $\frac{1}{8}$ inch and $\frac{1}{4}$ inch thicknesses. This pink felt is extra thick, and compared to moleskin, provides extra cushioning and a stronger adhesive base. Check with your local drugstore, medical supply store, or podiatrist for availability. **Hapad Inc.** is a mail-order source for adhesive surgical felt made from a rayon and wool blend in a roll $\frac{1}{4}$ inch thick by 6 inches by $7\frac{1}{2}$ feet. **Hapad Inc., (800) 544-2723, www.hapad.com**

BRAVE SOLDIER WOUND HEALING OINTMENT was formulated for athletes and is popular among cyclists. Developed by a dermatologist to keep abrasion wounds moist and protected, Brave Soldier helps heal blisters, road rash, minor cuts, and burns. It's made with tea tree oil as a natural antiseptic, aloe gel for its natural healing properties, jojoba oil as a natural moisturizer, vitamin E to rebuild collagen and skin tissue, shark liver oil to reduce scarring, and comfrey to stimulate skin cell growth and wound resurfacing. **Brave Soldier, (888) 711-BRAVE, www.bravesoldier.com**

MOLESKIN is a soft, cotton padding that protects skin surfaces against friction and has an adhesive backing that adheres to the skin. Dr. Scholl's makes Moleskin Plus from thin cotton-flannel padding and Moleskin Foam from soft latex foam. Moleskin is available in a variety of sizes in most drugstores, and it can be cut to the size needed. Hapad (see above) offers moleskin in a roll $\frac{1}{8}$ inch thick by 6 inches by $7\frac{1}{2}$ feet. Moleskin should not be applied directly over a blister because it can tear any loose skin when removed.

SPENCO PRESSURE PADS are made from closed-cell polyethylene foam that is soft, flexible, and thin. It is available in a six-pack of 3-by-5-inch sheets with two precut pads in ovals and circles and two uncut pads to be used over hot spots and blisters. **Spenco Medical Corporation, (800) 877-3626, www.spenco.com**

Advanced Blister Care

Even though the time-honored blister-care products are still used by many, there are more efficient products to both prevent blisters and promote healing. The chapter "Taping for Blisters" contains information that can be used as treatments for blisters. By following the methods described, you can apply tape over a blister whether the blister roof is intact or not. You can also apply tape can over Spenco 2nd Skin or other blister-care products mentioned below.

Tincture of benzoin applied to the area around a hot spot or blister will help blister products or tapes stick to the skin more effectively. Avoid getting tincture into a ruptured blister or other broken skin. After the tincture has dried, apply one of the blister-care products below. Be sure to apply a light coating of powder or lubricant to counteract the still exposed tincture of benzoin to prevent socks or contaminants from sticking to the skin. Be forewarned that forgetting this step when using tincture of benzoin on the toes may result in blisters from two toes being stuck together.

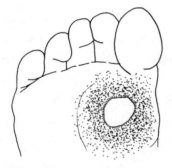 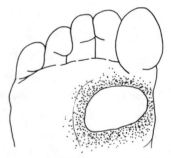

Tincture of benzoin (or any taping adherent) applied around a blister helps protective layers to adhere.

Once the protective coating covers the blister, apply a light coating of powder or lubricant to exposed benzoin.

Long-distance hiker and ultrarunner Brick Robbins uses tincture of benzoin around his blisters and then applies a Blister Relief pad. The pad usually will stay on for three to five days before falling off. After dealing with massive blisters, Steve Benjamin learned to use a Blister Relief pad placed over each area prone to blistering, overlapping them where necessary. He then puts tape over the Blister Relief pads to hold them in place. Using five pads per foot, he has eliminated his blister problem. This type of trial and error can be done with any blister prevention products. Scott Weber wraps the strips around his little toes to protect their blister-prone bottoms. Scott also uses Elastikon tape to anchor the pads to his forefeet. One runner uses a small Blister Relief on her toes, covers them with a Toe Cot (a latex rubber sheath), and then cuts off the extra Toe Cot and tapes the end.

There are several types of blister patches. Spenco 2nd Skin requires tape or a wrap to hold it in place. Spyroflex is adhesive but will stay in place better with tape over it. Xeroform is a yellowish petrolatum gauze dressing that can be cut and placed over a blister and then taped over. A small piece of 2nd Skin or DuoDerm can be cut to fill an open blister and then covered with tape over the top. This allows a runner to continue with little pain. It's the fluid in the blister that causes the pain.

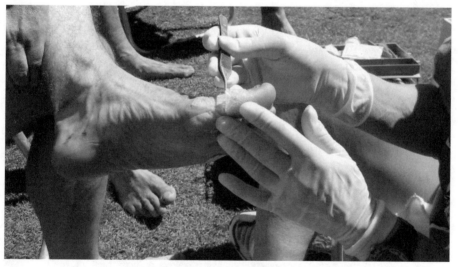

Applying 2nd Skin to blister.

U.S. Army Captain Dave Hamilton, a physician's assistant, learned a few tricks about how to treat blisters from Dutch Red Cross workers at the military Nijmegen 4-Day 140km March. Dave personally had this method used on his blistered feet after which he marched 25 and 26 miles respectively over two days with a 25- to 40-pound pack, wearing standard military boots. The

Dutch Red Cross method of taping feet over blisters is described in the chapter "Taping for Blisters." Here are their steps for dressing a blister:

1. Clean the blister area with an alcohol wipe.

2. Puncture blisters with a standard finger lancet (of the sort used in hospitals and blood banks to draw a few drops of blood).

3. Use the stick portion of a Q-Tip in a rolling motion to force the fluid out of a blister.

4. If the blister's roof has torn or is partially missing, trim off any loose edges.

5. If the blister is infected with pus, remove the roof of the blister and clean the blister cavity.

6. Cut a piece of DuoDerm in the shape and size of the open blister. Warm it in your gloved hands for 5 minutes to make it soft. Peel off the backing and place it inside the blister cavity. This forms an airtight dressing, soothes the wound, and fills the empty space inside the blister.

7. Tape over the patched blister.

If you have toe hot spots or blisters, you can use a gel toe cap to protect the whole toe. The caps are either solid gel or a fabric with gel inside. Bunga Toe Caps, Bunhead's Jelly Toes, Hapad's PediFix Visco-Gel Toe Caps, and Pro-Tec's Toe Caps are examples of these caps. With care these caps can be washed and reused.

TIP: Integrity Check

When using any of the products listed below on your blisters, be sure to occasionally check them. They may peel off, shift their position, or ball up under the stresses of hiking and running. When doing hills, the constant uphill and downhill movements of the feet combined with the pressures of the running body or the weight of a backpack may compromise their integrity. If you sense a change in how they feel, stop and check it out.

Instead of putting something on your feet, you can put ENGO Performance Patches inside your shoe or on your insole. These thin fabric-film composite patches can greatly reduce friction in targeted locations within your footwear by giving a slick, slippery surface to the area of your footwear or insole where friction is a problem.

ADVANCED BLISTER-CARE PRODUCTS

BAND-AID BLISTER RELIEF (formerly Compeed) is a blister cushion made with an elastic polyurethane film over a moisture absorbing and adhering layer, both covered with protective silicone papers that are removed for use. Functioning like a second layer of skin, Blister Relief cushions the area, virtually eliminating blister pain, while protecting it from further damage caused by friction. Tapered edges help adherence to the skin without rolling. It is not meant to be cut and can be worn for several days. For larger blisters, put two pieces side by side. Be careful not to wrinkle the edges of the pads. Blister Relief's hydrocolloid construction creates optimum conditions for rapid healing, while embedded cellulose particles absorb excess fluid and perspiration from the wound surfaces. Additionally, bacteria are sealed out, reducing the risk of infection. These pads can be left on until they come off on their own. Blister Relief comes in two sizes (a $^3/_4$-by-2 $^1/_4$-inch strip and a 1 $^5/_8$-by-2 $^5/_8$-inch oval), which are available in plastic compacts with either four (oval) or five (strips) pieces. Look for Blister Relief at drugstores, and running and sports stores. Band-Aid Blister Relief is made by **Johnson & Johnson**.

BUNGA TOE PADS AND TOE CAPS are made from a medical-grade polymer material. **Absolute Athletics, (888) 286-4272, www.bungapads.com**

BUNHEAD GEL products are made of a nonsilicone polymer, formulated with medical-grade mineral oils to cushion and protect those areas of the foot prone to friction trauma. They are washable, supple, comforting, hypoallergenic, nontoxic, dermatologist-tested, and cost-effective. The gel doesn't migrate, so it won't bottom out. The Jelly Tips, Jelly Toes, the Big Tip, and the really Big Tip are designed specifically for toes. Available at local retailers. **www.bunheads.com**

ADVANCED BLISTER-CARE PRODUCTS

COBAN is a self-adherent wrap that can be used around feet, ankles, and heels to hold blister products in place. Its elasticity and flexibility allows movement of the joints. Since it adheres to itself, it contains no adhesive. Because it is elastic, be careful not to apply it too tightly and cause constriction. Your pharmacy or medical supply stores typically carry Coban or similar self-adherent wraps. Most are available in 2-, 3-, and 4-inch widths.

DR. SCHOLL'S BLISTER TREATMENT sterile pads prevent blisters and help protect existing sores from pressure and abrasion. Cushlin pads adhere directly to skin, forming a tight seal around blisters. **Available at most drugstores.**

DUODERM CGF FLEXIBLE STERILE DRESSING is a polymer wound dressing used in hospitals. Packaged in a 4-by-4-inch size, it can be cut to fill the space inside an open blister. Buy the borderless dressings. **Available in medical supply stores or at Internet stores.**

ENGO PERFORMANCE PATCHES are made of a thin fabric-film composite that can greatly reduce friction in targeted locations within your footwear. The patches give a slick, slippery surface to the area of your footwear or insole where friction is a problem. The adhesive creates a strong bond, eliminating migration, even through moisture and sweat. When used for hot spots, blister formation is prevented. If used to help treat a blister, healing time is significantly decreased. Patches come in three sizes (small ovals, large ovals, and sheets), and they can be trimmed for a custom fit. The slippery blue top layer also acts as a change-out indicator, changing from blue to white as it wears through. Each patch is extremely durable, lasting anywhere from several weeks to several months. **Tamarack Habilitation Technologies Inc., (763) 795-0057, www.goengo.com**

HAPAD offers PediFix Visco-Gel Toe Caps that can be used over toe blisters. **Hapad Inc., (800) 544-2723, www.hapad.com**

MUELLER'S MORE SKIN pads have the feel and consistency of human skin and remove friction between two moving surfaces. More Skin is available in 3-inch circles, 1-inch circles and squares, and 3-inch squares. **Mueller Sports Medicine, Inc., (800) 356-9522, www.muellersportsmed.com**

ADVANCED BLISTER-CARE PRODUCTS

NEW-SKIN comes in two forms: a Liquid Bandage useful as a skin protectant or toughener, and a Wound & Blister Dressing. The Liquid Bandage, in a spray or liquid, dries rapidly to form a tough protective cover that is antiseptic, flexible, and waterproof, and it lets the skin breathe. The Wound & Blister Dressing comes in 2-inch squares. Look for New-Skin at drugstores.

PRO-TEC'S TOE CAPS, made from custom-grade silicone, are soft and stretchable to fit all toes. Locate a reseller through their Website. **www.pro-tec athletics.com**

SPENCO ADHESIVE KNIT can be used to cover 2nd Skin pads or as a skin protector to prevent blisters. Spenco Adhesive Knit is a highly breathable woven fiber with the ability to stretch and conform, and it does not come off from sweat or bathing. It cuts to size and fits easily around toes and hard to tape areas. Adhesive Knit comes in 3-by-5-inch rectangles in a six-pack. **Spenco Medical Corporation, (800) 877-3626, www.spenco.com**

SPENCO 2ND SKIN BLISTER PADS should be applied directly over blisters. Made with the 2nd Skin hydrocolloid pad bordered with a thin adhesive film, the pads keep blisters from drying out, absorb moisture and perspiration, and promote a scab free, naturally healed blister. Pads are 60mm by 45mm in an oval shape. Contact Spenco as listed above.

SPENCO 2ND SKIN DRESSINGS are unique skinlike hydrogel pads that can be applied directly over closed or open blisters. The pads help reduce friction and the discomfort of blisters. They can also be used over abrasions, cuts, or similar wounds. Use one or more pads to cover the blister area. Remove the cellophane layer on one side of the pad, apply that gel side to the blister, and then remove the cellophane from the other side. The pads do not stick to the skin and require tape to hold them onto the skin. They should be kept moist and changed daily. Cover the 2nd Skin pads with either Spenco Adhesive Knit, one of the tapes mentioned, moleskin, or a self-adhering wrap. These pads are available in a variety of sizes: 1-inch squares, 3-inch circles, and 3-by-6$\frac{1}{2}$-inch rectangles. Some sizes are nonsterile; others are sold as sterile Moist Burn Pads. Be sure to keep your packet of pads moist or they will dry out. Contact Spenco as listed above.

ADVANCED BLISTER-CARE PRODUCTS

SPYROFLEX is an adhesive wound dressing. It consists of a thin two-layered polyurethane membrane that has an adhesive inner side that goes against the skin and an outer layer that is moisture-vapor–permeable and microporous. As an "intelligent" dressing, Syproflex is open-cell, designed for moisture management. It helps protect the blister from external moisture and bacteria while speeding the healing process. Moisture from the blister is absorbed by the porous membrane, passes through, and evaporates. The pad, cut to size, is applied directly over the blister and may be left on for up to seven days, yet it is easily removed without sticking or tearing. Spyroflex works extremely well on inflamed and infected blisters. For maximum adherence, use as much of the pad as possible on the skin around the blister and cover the pad with Spenco Adhesive Knit or a similar porous tape. Spyroflex is available in an Abrasion Dressing Kit with three 4-inch square pads, a Blister Dressing Kit with five 2-inch square pads, and a Skin Savers package with eight pads in the two different sizes. All pads may be cut to size. **Outdoor Rx, (800) 531-5731, www.outdoorrx.com**

XEROFORM PETROLATUM GAUZE DRESSING is a sterile, nonadherent fine mesh gauze wound dressing. This product can be used over blisters. Xeroform is packaged in a 1-by-8-inch strip, a 5-by-9-inch rectangle, or a 4-inch-by-3-yard roll (for medical crews). It can be found in medical supply stores or Internet stores.

Extreme Blister Prevention & Care

Some athletes may choose to use extreme methods to initially prevent blisters or subsequently treat their blisters in order to continue on in a competitive event. These are aggressive methods. A competitive 100-mile, 24-hour, 48-hour, or six-day run may motivate a runner to want to try any means to keep running. Likewise, hikers may need to deal aggressively with blisters when in the middle of a multiday hike. The team participation rule in an adventure-racing event may force a team member to consider treating blisters in an extreme method.

There are several extreme methods for extreme blister prevention and care. Review the following methods to determine whether one may be useful for you in your running and hiking adventures.

The first extreme method is covered in the chapter "Taping for Blisters" (page 102). It can be used as an aggres-

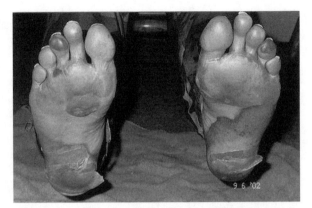

Under extreme conditions, entire feet can blister and whole skin layers can separate. It's best to do all you can to prevent such dire circumstances.

sive treatment for both blister prevention and treatment. By following the methods described in that chapter, tape can be applied over a blister, whether the blister roof is intact or not.

The second extreme method of blister prevention uses tincture of benzoin, or a similar benzoin-based product, and silicone cream. Marv Skagerberg still likes his benzoin and silicone-cream combination that worked for him for the last 78 of 86 days of the 1985 crosscountry Trans America race. Averaging 43 miles per day through 12 states, Marv did not get a single blister with the following method:

1. Clean the feet thoroughly, and dry them completely.

2. Coat the feet, heels, soles, and toes with tincture of benzoin.

3. Let the feet dry for 3 minutes, keeping the toes spread. The feet will still be quite sticky.

4. Apply a silicone cream. He uses Avon's Silicone Glove, which comes in a 1½-oz tube and is available through an Avon sales representative.

5. Put on a lightweight double-layer sock.

6. Reapply the cream every four to six hours and change socks at the same time.

Bill Trolan, MD, uses Hydropel Sports Ointment over Cramer's Tuf-Skin in the same manner as Marvin described above. He recommends reapplying Tuf-Skin, or similar benzoin product, and cream at every sock change. Many adventure racers swear by Hydropel because of it moisture repelling properties. Never underestimate the creative search for blister preventing ideas. Some athletes have found Sno-Seal Original Beeswax Waterproofing to be effective when applied over tincture of benzoin. Remember that any of these products needs to be reapplied when changing socks or every four to six hours when on your feet.

Dr. Trolan has participated in several Raid Gaulloises and served as a medical consultant to adventure-racing teams in the EcoChallenge as well as to Naval Special Warfare. He describes two more extreme methods of treating blisters, warning that they are "not for the faint of heart."[24] These treatments have helped many adventure racers finish their events. The methods should not be used if the blister is infected. Likewise, the following technique with tincture of benzoin can lead to infections and should ONLY be used if you accept the possible consequences. Permanent damage to the skin surfaces can occur.

After you have opened the blister and drained it thoroughly, and your feet are dry, use one of the following methods to seal down the blister roof:

- Use a syringe, without a needle, to inject tincture of benzoin directly into the blister. Immediately apply pressure across the top of the blister to evenly seal down the blister's outer layer to the underlying skin. This also pushes out any extra benzoin. Be forewarned that injecting the benzoin is momentarily painful. Dr. Trolan rates it as an eight on a one to ten pain scale where "childbirth and kidney stones are a ten and a paper cut is a one."

- Use New-Skin Liquid Bandage, instead of benzoin, injected into the blister. This does not seal the blister as well nor as long as benzoin, but it is less painful. Dr. Trolan rates it as a five or six on the pain scale.

At the 1996 Western States 100-Mile Endurance Run, Teresa Krall found out the hard way how painful tincture in a blister can be. The cotton ball used to apply the tincture was dropped into the dirt and one of her crew mistakenly decided to pour the tincture directly onto her blistered heel. As Brick Robbins, her pacer, recalls, "The tincture of benzoin was poured before I could object, followed by a blood curdling scream. After a while (it seemed like forever), Teresa quit screaming." Teresa recalls the blister being about half-dollar size and the pain being intense. She would not do it again unless it was the only method left to let her run; she would try Blister Relief first.

Using Syringes & Needles

You may see medical aid station people using syringes with needles to draw out the blister fluid and then to inject the tincture. Syringes with needles must be sterile in order to prevent infection. There is no safe way to dispose of the syringes and needles, or "sharps" as they are called in the medical profession, except in a sharps container. If you use syringes and needles outside of a medical station, store the sharps in a hard-shelled container until they can be safely disposed of.

In this time of hepatitis, HIV, and AIDS, we need to practice universal precautions—in this case, hand washing and switching to new gloves before treating each person. An open blister must be treated as an open wound, and the blister's fluid must be treated as a bodily fluid. Additionally, there is a danger that using a syringe you might inject more tincture than is necessary to get a good seal or not enough to cover all inner surfaces. By making several small puncture holes in the blister, and using a syringe without a needle, excess tincture can be pushed out when pressure is applied to the roof of the blister. A good seal is then ensured.

George Freelen, a former Army Ranger, recalls how when he was in the army, he used the tincture to seal blisters. He vividly remembers "it hurts like hell, but only for 15 to 20 seconds." This method is no longer taught or accepted in the army. The choice is yours. It works to seal the blister's roof to the inner skin so running and hiking can continue. But there is definitely pain and always the risk of infection, and other treatments are available.

After sealing the blister, Dr. Trolan suggests several options. Apply a coating of tincture of benzoin to help the tape or moleskin better adhere to the skin. Or apply Instant Krazy Glue over the blister. This layer provides an extra layer of protection and helps your tape covering better adhere to the skin. *Do not use Krazy Glue in the blister.*

For severe cases, Dr. Trolan has used the tincture of benzoin injection, followed by a coating of tincture of benzoin on top of the blister, followed by a coating of New-Skin Liquid Bandage, followed by a layer of Krazy Glue, and finally followed by tape or moleskin. He recommends using an emery board or fine nail file to smooth any rough spots on the blister coating before applying tape or moleskin.

Ultrarunner and former Appalachian Trail record holder David Horton recommends using the combination of antibiotic and drying-agent zinc oxide on blisters when you have an overnight stop or a rest period for the zinc oxide to do its magic. He remembers using the zinc-oxide method on blisters when running the Trans-America (across the United States). He advises that you "take a needle and drain the blister. Then using the same hole, inject zinc oxide back into the blister until it is full of zinc. Put a Band-Aid over that. Many times we would do that in the Trans-Am and the next day the blister would be nearly dried up. It is still the best thing I have seen to do to a blister." David made this blister fix one time on ultrarunner Dusan Marjele, the eventual Trans-Am winner, and he came back several more times because it was so effective.

In the March 2001 issue of *Men's Health* magazine, Chris Patrick, a former trainer at the University of Florida, also promoted the use of zinc oxide. He suggests squeezing it directly into a blister after draining the fluid out. He makes another suggestion for when large areas of skin were lost from blisters: pack the wound with cornstarch, which dries out the area and hardens. Over the cornstarch he sprays Tuff Skin. He admits this "stings like hell."

personal experience

"Leukotape rocks! This was the best tape. Unfortunately, [at the Primal Quest Race] we had only one roll and went through it quickly. The adhesive was far superior to any other we had available and the tape shaped well to toes and feet.

"For blisters that were open with macerated or infected tissue, we used Xeroform gauze. This is the petrolatum and antiseptic impregnated bandage that is often used for sucking chest wounds. It worked particularly well for blisters in between the toes. We cut the gauze pads to size and wrapped them around the toes and then taped over them. Unfortunately, we could not talk to the racers at the end to see how well this worked, but it seemed like a good idea.

"We used syringe needles (mostly 18-gauge) to drain the blisters. The larger size needle allowed the fluid to drain easily through the needle, without risk of it closing back up. Some also used the bevel edge to cut a slightly larger opening. We drained any blisters, large or small, that had palpable fluid. To clip or not to clip blister was on a case-by-case basis. We never clipped intact blisters, but open or torn skin was often removed to prevent further tearing.

"If the area was tender, we taped it. Any reddened or sore area was either taped or covered with moleskin. If the racers had done this earlier, I think we would have seen fewer patients.

"A podiatrist showed us a trick to keep tape from curling at the edges. She takes a normal votive candle and, after taping, rubs it over the edges of the tape. The small amount of wax reduces friction and helps prevent curling. This is less messy than using Bag Balm or Vaseline.

"Two people had infected cuticles due to ingrown toenails. The doctor had to lift the cuticle and drain the pus. Obviously, these racers didn't read John's book on trimming your toenails!"

—Adventure racer and paramedic Jane Moorhead, relating how her medical crew managed feet in the 2003 Subaru Primal Quest Adventure Race

Deep Blisters

Usually the only way to treat deep blisters is to use a syringe and needle to drain the fluid. The blister is so deep that nothing else can get in that deep. The athlete knows there is a blister there—but it is almost impossible to drain. Pressing on the callus to try to expel the fluid by hand is too painful. Using a pin or scalpel won't work. Only in the biggest races with a full medical staff will there likely be a doctor who has the Zylocaine and equipment to properly care for these blisters.

Read the section on calluses (below) to understand how to soften these problem areas. It is true that many athletes value their toughened feet and calluses. For some, they help. For others, they mask hidden deep blisters.

personal experience

"Deep blisters are next to impossible to treat. I can think of one instance in which a runner used a combination of tincture of benzoin and Hydropel in combination to do a Badwater double. He got through the one way to the top of Mt. Whitney, but his feet were a mess by the time he was ready to do the return trip. You see, he didn't want to bother with pretaping. I don't blame him; it's a time-consuming effort to do it. But he developed blisters so deep on his heels and the balls of his feet that he could not move forward. They became blood blisters. My husband, Ben Jones, who is a medical doctor, injected him with Zylocaine, so that the blisters could be drained and treated. Under normal race circumstances it's impossible to get an injection to drain blisters. Usually there isn't that resource in a race.

"That is why I recommend filing calluses down so that if one develops a blister on that area it can be drained and treated. Otherwise, [the blister] just grows and it becomes impossible to move forward. Once the fluid is drained, the blister is treated with antibiotic ointment and 2nd Skin, and taped. It's then possible to keep on moving quite comfortably."

—Denise Jones, the Blister Queen of Badwater

Beyond Blisters

There may be times when blisters develop and even with treatment, due to continued running or hiking, additional care is needed. Several things may happen. The skin may slough off and ball up in the sock, leaving raw exposed skin. The skin may stay in place but fall off when the sock is removed. The raw skin may bleed. When blisters have developed to this point, you have to make a a choice. Continuing to run or hike may lead to infection. Ideally, stay off the feet as much as possible. If you must continue, treat the problem and recheck frequently.

Sterile wound-dressing products will help the healing process. Medical personnel should have several of these products in their kits to manage extreme blisters and cases where the skin has separated from the foot. These dressings are typically available only through medical supply stores but may also be found through an Internet search:

- Convatec's DuoDerm CGF Flexible Sterile Dressing (4 by 4 inch)
- Cramer Products' Nova Derm (4 by 4 inch and 3 by 6 inch, glycerine gel formula)
- Mueller Sports Medicine's Dermal Pads (4 by 4 inch, closed-cell elastomer)
- Spenco's 2nd Skin Moist Burn Pads (1½ by 2 inch, 2 by 3 inch, and 3 by 4 inch, thin gel sheets)
- Spyroflex's square pads (2 inch and 4 inch)

Use these products over the blister or raw skin and leave them on as the healing process begins from the inside. The nonadhesive dressings require a tape covering or self-adhering wrap to hold them in place. One of these carried on a multiday hike could easily save one's feet.

Fixing Blisters, Their Way or Yours

You may find yourself entering in an event in which you do not have control over the blister treatments and how they are applied. Participate in a 100-mile trail event or an EcoChallenge, and you will find medical aid stations manned by podiatrists, podiatry students, nurses, emergency medical technicians, and an assortment of individuals with various medical skills. These individuals will treat your blisters according to what they know and what materials they have available to them. How they treat your blisters may not be how you would like them treated. Most aid stations are stocked with moleskin, Vaseline, and gauze. They may or may not have 2nd Skin, alcohol wipes, and tincture of benzoin. If you want your feet treated with Blister Relief, 2nd Skin, or another product, you will have to carry a few pieces of these in your fanny pack. If you want a specific powder or lubricant you will need to carry these in a small container.

For example, the Marathon des Sables is unlike any other marathon or ultramarathon. The six-day, self-supported race in the Moroccan desert has 150 miles of sand, sand, and more sand. Cathy Tibbetts-Witkes, a many-time Marathon des Sables finisher, calls it a blisterfest: "Even people who never get blisters get them." While the medical care is adequate and very good, it is not everyone's first choice of blister care. Cathy reports the usual procedure is to lance the blisters, cut the skin off, apply tincture of benzoin, and then apply Compeed. While this is not my first choice of treatment, it does work. Runners report a low incident of infection despite the high level of open blisters. Remember: a lack of preparedness on your part means you will be treated as the medical team has been taught.

Dr. Trolan stresses the importance of understanding how your feet change when you add things to them. Adding moleskin and gauze to your foot changes the way your foot fits inside your shoe or boot. The extra thickness of the blister patch changes pressures and angles of the foot inside the shoe. This in turn changes the shoe from its usually "broken-in" fit to that of a "mismatch." New pressure points develop, turning first into new hot spots and then into blisters. The biomechanics of the foot and ankle and leg are altered and the gait changes. Additional problems are likely to develop. Dr. Trolan recommends using as little and as thin a blister patch as possible.

Do not hesitate to give medical personnel at these aid stations instruction on how you would like your feet patched. I remember the bulky gauze patch put on the bottom of my right foot in 1986 during the final stages of my first Western States 100-Mile Endurance Run. While it was a good patch job, it simply did not fit right and turned me from a runner into a walker. Be aware of how medical staff are treating your feet. If you prefer a specific method of blister patching, you need to tell them, and be prepared to describe it to them.

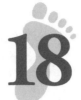

18

Strains & Sprains, Fractures & Dislocations

Ankle sprains and strains are common occurrences—some even with resulting fractures. Bones can break as a result of falls or twisting motions, and stress fractures can occur if athletes push themselves too fast and too soon, an unfortunately common tendency. A sudden fall with its resulting wrong landing can result in a dislocated ankle or toe. The cause may be rocks or tree roots hidden in leaves or grasses, unsteady footing while trail running at night, or twisting motions coming off a curb. Athletes need to be prepared to deal with these injuries quickly and appropriately, as late or inadequate treatment can worsen the injury, sidelining you longer and possibly setting you up for future injuries.

Strains & Sprains

A *strain* is the overstretching of a muscle or tendon—but without the significant tearing common to a sprain. There may be bleeding into the muscle area that can cause swelling, pain, stiffness, and muscle spasm followed by a bruise. Strains can come from overuse, repetitive movements, excessive muscle contractions, or prolonged positions.

A *sprain* is a stretching or tearing injury to the ligaments that stabilize bones together at a joint. Sprains are usually associated with traumas such as falling or twisting, and ankles are frequently the sprained or strained joint. During a fall or sudden twist, you may experience sudden pain or hear a pop. If you cannot walk after a few minutes of rest or if you heard the infamous "pop," you can be fairly certain you have a sprain. After a sprain occurs, the fibrous joint capsule swells and becomes inflamed, discolored, and painful. An X-ray is in order. Delaying treatment for sprains or strains increases the risk of swelling and further injury. One ankle sprain will make you more susceptible to repeated sprains, as the ligaments are left weakened, lengthened, and less flexible.

Ultrarunner Sue Norwood calls herself the "queen of ankle sprains." She shares this advice: "I have learned from my 22 years of experience as a patient with recurring ankle problems from trail running. My ankle sprains got progressively worse until I ruptured two peroneal tendons in one ankle and had to have surgery to reattach them. It's better to learn effective preventive techniques than letting yourself get this injured!"

The most common ankle sprain is an "inversion" sprain, in which the foot rolls to the outside and the ankle turns out. The injured area is the lateral ligament just below the ankle joint on the outside of the foot. An "eversion" sprain, in which the ankle is turned inward and the medial ligament injured, is less common. In a serious sprain, both the lateral and medial ligaments can be injured. An X-ray will reveal whether there is a bone fracture that would require immobilization of the joint.

There are three degrees of an ankle sprain. A grade 1 strain has minimal swelling, and the athlete can still put weight on the leg with the twisted ankle. The ankle's ligaments have been stretched and some are torn. A grade 2 sprain has moderate swelling and moderate pain when weight is put on the injured ankle. There is a partial tear of the ligament. A grade 3 sprain has a large amount of swelling, and weight placed on the ankle cannot be tolerated. Grades 1 and 2 will heal in about four to six weeks with full recovery in 10 to 12 weeks.

A grade 3 sprain requires medical attention. With a severe sprain there is the possibility of a related fracture. If there is a great deal of pain and swelling, and you are unable to bear weight on the foot, an emergency room visit and an X-ray are in order.

There are ways to minimize ankle sprains. Obvious but often forgotten, specific strengthening exercises can go a long toward preventing strains and sprains (see "Strengthening Exercises," page 234). In addition, always be aware of how your feet land. If you sense your foot starting to roll over, quickly transfer your weight to your other foot. When on the trail, be attentive to changes in the terrain, especially on downhills and in the late afternoon and evenings when shadows merge into darkness. On the road, be aware of curbs, manholes, and grates, and the slanted, concave surface roadway. On grassy areas, watch for hidden holes and roots. Any of these can trip you up and throw you off balance. Additionally, you are more susceptible to making wrong moves and being slower to respond to sudden terrain changes when you are tired.

Treating a Strain or Sprain

The initial treatment for a strain or sprain includes the classic RICE treatment:

- R = rest
- I = ice
- C = compression
- E = elevation

Ice your injury within 30 minutes if possible. The first 24 hours are the most critical for beginning treatment. The typical sprained ankle takes four to six weeks to fully heal. Severe ankle sprains can require a cast for complete immobilization.

Early treatment within the first 24 hours decreases swelling and lessens the risk of additional injury. Initial rest of the foot is also important. A lightly applied Ace wrap will provide compression to help keep swelling down while providing support. Apply the Ace wrap from the forefoot towards the ankle. Do not wear the Ace wrap at night. Apply ice for 20 minutes at a time at least four times daily. The chapter "Cold & Heat Therapy" gives more information on making the most of icing techniques.

Elevate the injured area above the level of the heart as much as possible during the first 48 hours. This keeps blood away from the injured area and reduces pain and swelling. In bed at night, elevate the foot on a pillow. The treatment goal is to return the ankle to normal motion and to be weight bearing as soon as possible. The combination of rest, icing, compression, and elevation, especially in the first few days, will help the healing process and decrease the pain and swelling.

Heat increases blood flow to an injured area, which makes swelling worse. For this reason, the use of heat is not recommended for at least a week after an injury. Moist heat can be applied by using a moist heating pad, a warm towel, or a warm bath. Dry heat can be applied by using a heating pad for 20 minutes at a time.

The use of anti-inflammatory medications is usually warranted. Nonsteroidal anti-inflammatory drugs, commonly called NSAIDS, are used to control pain and swelling after an injury. The most common NSAIDS are aspirin, ibuprofen, and naproxen sodium (Aleve). These pain relievers should be taken according to their instructions and usually with food. Be careful if you continue training because the NSAIDS block pain signals that would warn you of further injury.

Depending on the severity of the injury, you might be able to walk on it. With minimal pain and swelling, self-treatment at home can often be sufficient. If the pain is severe with a large degree of swelling and there is discoloration of the injured area, prompt medical attention is mandatory.

There are two schools of thought on how soon to start running, exercising, or bearing weight on an injured ankle. The one says to get out on it as soon as possible and let pain be your guide. If the ankle is stiff and sore when you first start, keep going and see if it loosens up. If the pain increases you should call it a day, go home and ice. If it doesn't get worse or feels better you are probably OK. The other says to work through the healing process at the ankle's speed. You must choose your course based on available information.

Certified athletic trainer Jay Hodde, MS, ATC/L, points out the following dangers of running too soon on an injured ankle:

Running with a severe sprain can cause more problems than just reinjuring it. Several things may happen. First, your gait will change as you guard the injury. Because your body is not used to these changes, overuse injuries may occur in other areas of the body. Second, the severity of the sprain may increase, prolonging recovery. Third, the ankle joint may develop the tendency to partially dislocate (subluxation). This is more common if the sprain is severe. Usually, there is some minor 'slipping' of bone surfaces that can cause problems if the joint mechanics are thrown off by the sprain. Bruising of the bone surfaces can occur and can lead to complications later in life, such as an increased risk of arthritis.

When you can start to put weight on the ankle, begin with easy walking and slowly build back to the routine you had before the injury. Wear an ankle support if you cannot bear your full weight on the ankle. Walking even a little bit a few times a day will aid on the road to recovery. After each exercise period, ice as necessary. Following a few of the strengthening exercises described below will also help you gain back ankle strength and normal motion.

Ankle supports are an important part of treating an ankle sprain or strain. The support will allow you to be up and about faster and will provide comfort as the ankle continues healing. There are many types to choose from. The section "Ankle-Support Products" (below) describes an assortment of available supports. But rather than becoming dependent on ankle supports, work on strengthening your ankles and sense of balance.

You can strengthen your ankles by focusing on *proprioception,* the neurological signals from your body to your brain that tell it where your body is relative to the space around it. Several exercises below focus on this aspect of ankle strengthening, which improves your ability to balance. Many athletes swear by proprioceptive reconditioning after an ankle injury. When you are able to make a midstride adjustment as your foot hit the ground, senses an uneven surface, and sends a signal to the brain, you are more likely to avoid a sprained ankle. The use of a wobble or rocker board is also helpful.

Josh Gilbert, a chiropractor, thinks a wobble or rocker board is a good tool. He suggests the following: "First, I would do a very simple activity. Stand on the injured ankle and balance for as long as you can. If you can do this for 30 seconds or longer, start doing the same exercise with your eyes closed. This helps to get your brain neurologically connected again with your ankle and the injured tissue and receptors. Only do this exercise if the ankle can bear your weight without pain (or not too much). Each joint in your body has receptors that tell your brain where it is. You don't have to look at your leg to know that it is turned in, out, pointed up, or down. The receptors in the joint relay this information to the brain. When the joint is injured, sprained, stretched, these receptors start relaying incorrect information. It they are not retrained properly, you will end up like many people and continue having recurrent ankle sprains."

Supplements for Quick Recovery

Since ligaments and tendons do not have their own direct blood supply, their healing is slow. Ultrarunner Karl King found that the nutritional supplements of 1g glycine, 1g lysine, 0.5g buffered vitamin C, and one Aleve tablet is helpful in the healing process. Take this combination at breakfast and at bedtime. The supplements provide the major building blocks for connective tissue, while the Aleve is an anti-inflammatory.

Two dietary supplements, glucosamine sulfate and chondroitin sulfate, have been found to reduce joint pain. Glucosamine sulfate is a natural substance that helps build cartilage, the cushion at the ends of our bones, and maintain joint fluid thickness and elasticity. Chondroitin sulfate, also a natural substance, helps lubricate joints and gives tendons and ligaments their elasticity. Initial studies have found these over-the-counter supplements helpful in stimulating cartilage to grow and inhibiting the enzymes that break down cartilage. Many athletes have added this combination to their daily vitamin and supplement intake as a "must have." Drugstores, pharmacies, and health food stores typically offer these two supplements (often in one capsule) in an assortment of supplement formulas by different companies. Give these supplements time to work—a month or more.

Strengthening Exercises

Strengthening exercises for the foot and ankle can help prevent injuries and can speed recovery from an injury. Balancing exercises are good to help strengthen the ankles. Stop any weight-bearing exercises if you experience pain. Here are some exercise options:

- Sit in a chair and write the alphabet with your toes to simulate ankle motion in all directions.
- Stand on one foot on a pillow or similar soft and unstable cushion and try to maintain your balance, first with one foot and then the

other. As your ability to balance increases, move into short controlled up and down knee bends.

■ Move the ankle up and down in a pumping motion to help decrease swelling.

■ Rotate your feet up to 50 repetitions in each direction. Do four to five sets every other day.

■ Strengthen your ankles by balancing with one foot flat on the ground and the other leg bent back at the knee, as if you were in the normal support phase of a running stride. Start at 30 seconds at a time and practice until you can hold your balance for several minutes. When you have mastered this step, close your eyes and do the same thing. Repeatedly losing your balance and then recovering gradually strengthens the ankles even more. Doing this exercise with your eyes closed retrains you to quickly react to changes as your nerve endings detect a twist or turn when the foot hits the ground. Mike Bate eliminated ankle problems by doing this one simple exercise.

■ Stand on one leg and slowly rise all the way up onto your toes and then slowly lower your heel to a flat foot. Balance yourself as necessary. Start with 25 repetitions and work up to 50 daily. This is another good proprioception exercise.

■ Stand with your forefeet on a raised surface (such as a book, low step, or block of wood), and rise up onto your toes and then back down again. Hold each, at the top and at the bottom, for 10 to 15 seconds. Repeat until both calves are fatigued.

■ An isometric exercise with the feet pushing against each other helps strengthen muscles without joint movement. When sitting on a chair, push down with one foot on top while pulling up with the other foot on the bottom. Then reverse feet. When sitting on the floor, you can also put your feet bottom-to-bottom, first pushing the big toes against each other and then the small toes against each other. Hold the motions for six to ten seconds and repeat several times a day.

■ Hop on one foot and then change to the other foot. Practice forward and backward, and side to side movements.

Work Those Calves

Matt Mahoney, one of the proponents of barefoot running and running without socks, feels the most important ankle muscle is the calf: "This is what you use to take the weight off your heel and shift to the ball of your foot when your ankle starts to twist." He recommends the following calf exercises, emphasizing, "You will know you're doing these exercises right if your calves are sore for several days afterwards."

- Run backwards.

- Run barefoot in sand.

- Climb stairs (on real stairs), both up and down. Land on the ball of your foot as you descend.

- Do calf raises on a step, with weights, standing for the gastrocnemius and sitting for the soleus. Using machines is useful for these. Do the standing calf raises one foot at a time on a step with a weighted belt. Do the sitting raises on a machine with weight resting on a padded bar across the top of the legs.

Ankle-Support Products

Weak ankles can be a problem, particularly on trails. After turning or spraining an ankle, an ankle support will provide the support and protection necessary for light training. Otherwise weak ankles can also benefit from an ankle support. Adhesive taping of the ankle can be helpful; however, for it to be effective, someone who is experienced must do the taping. While taping restricts extreme motion, the tape loses strength as it moves with the skin—40 percent of its strength can be lost within 20 minutes.

Ankle supports are typically made from a compression type sock. Some offer a figure-eight–style stretch wrap, which gives additional strength and support. Some ankle supports can be found in drugstores and sporting-goods stores. Cramer, Futuro, Mueller, Pro-Tec, and Spenco all make basic ankle supports. Many are simply a one-piece pull-on neoprene or stretch device with a hole for the heel and toes. Ace wraps, or similar elastic wraps, are helpful after a sprain but provide little support against initially turning your ankle. Sue Norwood, who has an eversion problem, likes the ASO

Ankle Stabilizer that her doctor told her to wear for the year after her surgery—it's supportive but lightweight and easy to use.

All the ankle supports listed below are compact in size and fit easily into a fanny pack or backpack. Since the supports vary in fit and material, experiment wearing the support against the skin or over a sock to find the best fit on your foot. If you are prone to ankle injuries, consider carrying one as a preventative measure.

ANKLE-SUPPORT PRODUCTS

The **ANKLE STABILIZING ORTHOSIS (ASO)** is made to prevent or treat ankle sprains. It features an elastic cuff closure to decrease the degree of potential inversion, figure-eight straps to replicate ankle taping, a low profile to allow it to fit in any type of shoe, and a lace-up closure. It is designed to keep the foot in a neutral position. A model is available with rigid side stays to increase stability. **Medical Specialties, (800) 582-4040, www.medspec.com**

The convenient **ANKLEWRAP** differs from the typical ACE wrap. Made from a knitted blend of nylon and Lycra with a foam inner layer, it breathes to wick away perspiration, stays put with superior sticking power, and is fully adjustable. At 10 feet long by $1\frac{1}{2}$ inches wide, it is long enough to make a complete figure-eight wrap with three heel locks. **Fabrifoam Products, (800) 577-1077, www.fabrifoam.com**

CHO-PAT'S ANKLE SUPPORT provides compression to the ankle with a removable Velcro fastener that wraps in a figure eight around the ankle giving additional compression at specific locations of the ankle while providing stabilization. The support is made of neoprene. **Cho-Pat, Inc., (800) 221-1601, www.cho-pat.com**

CROPPER MEDICAL'S BIO SKIN is a compression support material made with four layers: a hypoallergenic Lycra knit outer layer, a SmartSkin membrane that absorbs moisture and wicks it from the skin, a Lycra knit/fleece inner layer, and a SkinLok layer against the skin. Bio Skin stretches with the body's movement, giving compression without bunching and binding, and it does not constrict the joints. Unlike neoprene, Bio Skin breathes. The three designs

ANKLE-SUPPORT PRODUCTS

include a TriLok Ankle Control System, a Visco Ankle Skin that has visco polymer inserts around anklebones, and a Standard Ankle Skin. The visco and standard wraps have an optional figure-eight wrap. **Cropper Medical, (800) 541-2455, www.bioskin.com**

The **KALLASSY ANKLE SUPPORT** is a proven design for rehabilitation of severe ankle sprains. The support is made of nylon-lined neoprene that provides warmth and compression. A strap that wraps around the ankle provides stability, and a nonstretch lateral strapping system helps prevent inversion motions of the ankle. If you are prone to turned ankles, this support is one of the most stabilizing ankle supports available. Distributed through Kimberly-Clark, it is often available in sporting-goods stores or can be purchased via the Internet.

The **PERFORM 8 LATERAL ANKLE STABILIZER** provides excellent external stabilization of the ankle's lateral (outer) ligaments, similar to ankle taping. While a lightweight elastic compression sock provides support to soft tissue, an elastic figure-eight configuration strap wraps around the foot. Pads protect and relieve pressure on the Achilles tendon. This support is excellent for athletes prone to chronic ankle sprains. **Brown Medical Industries, (800) 843-4395, www.brownmed.com**

STROMGREN makes several ankle supports that provide good stabilization to prevent turning an ankle or to support a previously sprained ankle. Their Double Strap Model offers a unique sock-style support with two elastic straps that wrap around the ankle to provide the benefit of taped ankle support without the tape. The Stirrup Lock Ankle Support has four straps that restrict inversion/eversion. **Stromgren Supports, (800) 430-3875, www.stromgren.com**

WOBBLE & ROCKER BOARDS can be used to improve balance and strength, retrain injured muscles, improve muscle memory, and build core strength. Fitter First has the most comprehensive line of boards, and training charts and programs. **Fitter International, (800) 348-8371, www.fitter1.com**

Fractures

Any bone in the foot can fracture: however, some are more prone to injury than others. The terms *break* and *fracture* are synonymous—both describe a structural break in the continuity of the bone. A fracture may occur from a fall, the twisting motion of a turned ankle, a blow from hitting your foot on a rock or tree root, or simply from a bad foot plant. The toes are most likely bones to fracture in the foot—usually the first (big toe) and the fifth (small toe). The Jones fracture (breaking the fifth metatarsal on the outside of the foot) is common. This type of fracture is common with a fall or loss of balance where you put a sudden and undue amount of pressure on the outside of your foot. But there are many types of fractures.

Types of Fractures

AVULSION—the tearing away of a part of the bone attached to a ligament or tendon.

BUTTERFLY—a bone fragment shaped like a butterfly and part of a comminuted fracture.

COMMINUTED—more than two fragments; may be splintered.

COMPLETE—the bone is completely broken through.

DISPLACED—bone fragments are moved away from each other.

IMPACTED—fragments are compressed by force into each other or adjacent bone.

INCOMPLETE—the continuity of the bone is destroyed on only one side.

NONDISPLACED—the bone pieces are still together in the correct locations/angles.

SEGMENTAL—several large fractures in the same bone.

SPIRAL—the fracture line is spiral in shape.

Fractures usually manifest themselves with a great deal of pain and tenderness directly above the fracture site. When a soft tissue injury has occurred, there will also be discoloration of the skin above the fracture. Fractures that are ignored can result in a malunion or nonunion of the pieces of bone as they heal. This could require surgery to correctly align the bone ends.

Emergency room physicians and sports specialists often use the Ottowa Ankle Rules[25] to determine the likelihood of an ankle fracture before an X-ray is taken (and to avoid unnecessary X-rays). The study takes two approaches:

- Pain in the malleolar (ankle bones) zone and either and inability to bear weight immediately and in the emergency room, or bone tenderness at the posterior (back) edge of either malleolus.

- Pain in the midfoot zone and either an inability to bear weight immediately and in the emergency room, or bone tenderness at the navicular (the bone at the top front of the foot at the curve up the ankle) or fifth metatarsal (the midfoot bone on the outside of the foot).

Treating Fractures

Treatment of fractures typical combines ice, immobilization, and elevation. Toe fractures are usually buddy taped, and the patient is advised to wear a firm-soled shoe or a wooden orthopedic shoe that restricts flexion of the foot. Buddy taping is done by lightly taping the injured toe to the toe next to it, with a piece of cotton between toes (never tape skin to skin). Buddy taping provides support and a limited degree of immobilization of the toe. A fracture of the big toe can warrant a full foot cast. A Jones fracture or any other fracture of the foot or ankle will require a cast and immobilization for between four to six weeks.

Standard practice with fractures is to immobilize the joint above and the joint below the fracture. You may start out with a nonweight-bearing cast, requiring the use of crutches, and later have it changed to a weight-bearing walking cast.

Refer to the chapter "Cold & Heat Therapy" (page 306) for more information on making the most of icing techniques.

Stress Fractures

Stress fractures are a common sports injury. Sudden or repetitive stress, usually from overuse without proper conditioning, results in a small crack in the outer shell of the affected bone. Over time, if not treated, this crack will develop into a fracture of the bone. Often you will no recollection of having injured the foot.

The most common foot bones to stress fracture are the second and third metatarsal bones in the forefoot—between the toes and the ankle. Some doctors will use an X-ray to make the diagnosis, but often a stress fracture does not show on an initial X-ray because the bone's callus formation has not yet taken place at the fracture site. A bone scan, which is different from an X-ray, is useful for a questionable diagnosis and will usually confirm whether you have a stress fracture. Some hospitals will use an MRI to make the diagnosis.

Other possible causes of stress fractures include wearing worn-out or poor-fitting shoes, or ill-fitting insoles; abnormal foot structure or mechanics (arch or pronation problems, or leg-length discrepancies); or tightness and inflexibility. Your medical specialist may recommend additional calcium in your diet and/or a DEXA scan bone-density test. Female athletes who have infrequent periods are most at risk for stress fractures.

At the point of the stress fracture, there is typically pain to the touch, often first felt as a dull ache or soreness. The pain usually becomes worse as the break grows. Swelling is common. Stress fractures are most common from overuse, over-training, or a change in running surfaces—from a softer to a harder surface. Stress fractures are also referred to as "march fractures."

Peter Fish's stress-fracture story is not so unusual. He remembers his first stress fracture (to the third metatarsal of the right foot), which happened in July 1995. His second fracture may have started as a stress fracture or may have simply been a fracture from the start:

> I had had an unpleasant "itchy" sensation on the top of my foot for a month or so (I was ramping up mileage for the Portland Marathon), and during a training run, it turned into a sudden sharp pain. I limped home and went to my family doctor the same day. The fracture didn't show on the X-ray yet, but it appeared a couple of weeks later when I consulted my podiatrist. I didn't use the walking boot,

but if I had to do a lot of walking, I found that a stiff-soled pair of medium-high work boots kept my foot from flexing painfully and enabled me to walk almost normally. I didn't run for six weeks, and then I started off cautiously, this time with the California International Marathon (early December) in mind.

This time my training went quite well, with no protests from the injured foot, and I was able to get up to 40 miles a week with five or six long runs. I ran two races during the month or so before the marathon, one of nine miles and the other a 20K, both at my projected marathon pace. A couple of weeks before the race, the top of my left foot felt sore. My podiatrist thought it was probably a neuroma from too tight laces, as it was rather high up on the instep for a stress fracture. I ran the marathon, in some discomfort, although this didn't seem to get worse during the race, and I managed to attain my Boston qualifier by a couple of minutes with a time of 3:38.

Immediately after the race, my foot became extremely painful, and I could hardly walk on it. It was a couple of weeks before I could run at all, and I had to run on the outside of that foot to do it. It didn't seem to be healing at all, so I went back to the podiatrist. An X-ray showed it to be fractured quite badly, nearly all the way through. The reason I could run on it was that the break was near the top of the third metatarsal, where there was less flexion. The doctor thought it seemed more like a break due to trauma than a normal stress fracture. During the nine-mile race I had run a couple of months previous, I got off the course once and had to jump a ditch to get back. I landed pretty heavily, and it seemed possible that this set up the fracture, which came on later, perhaps during the marathon. The regimen was the same as before: no running for six weeks, and as before, I spent a lot of time in the pool, on my bike, and even did some cross-country skiing.

Treating Stress Fractures

After a confirming scan, a sports doctor, orthopedist, or podiatrist will usually recommend at least six weeks off. Follow their advice. To run or exercise heavily on a stress fracture is asking for more problems. Switch to more cushioned shoes and use this recovery time to focus on other nonweight-bearing exercises and cross-training: cycling, pool running, swimming, and weight training. Ask your doctor whether you can use a limited-weight–bearing exercise machine like a stair climber or elliptical trainer.

An Ace wrap or compression sock will help control swelling. An orthopedic or wooden shoe may be used to splint the foot. Anti-inflammatories are helpful. Elevation of the foot above the level of the heart will help reduce pain and swelling. Ice the area 20 minutes at a time three to four times a day and after any exercise. The "Cold & Heat Therapy" chapter gives more information on making the most of icing techniques. Difficult cases may require splinting, casting, or surgery.

Dislocations

A *dislocation* is a complete displacement of bone from its normal position at a joint's surface, which disrupts the articulation of two or three bones at that junction and alters alignment. The dislocation may be complete, where the joint surfaces are completely separated, or incomplete (subluxation), where the joint is only slightly displaced. The dislocation may be caused by a direct blow or injury, or by a ligament's tearing.

In the foot, the most common dislocations are the toes. Any of the toes can be dislocated, but the most typical are the big toe or the small toe. The ankle can be dislocated by any combination of fractures of the tibia (the big inner bone of the lower leg) or fibula (the small outer bone of the lower leg), resulting in a displaced talus. Ankle dislocations can be a major lower leg injury with severe consequences if the circulation to the foot is compromised.

Treating Dislocations

Dislocated toes are fairly simple to treat. Resetting dislocations is called *reduction*. With one hand, stabilize the ball of the foot with your thumb on the injured toe. With the other hand exert traction to the toe while pulling slowly and steadily on the displaced section of toe. Pull firmly enough that it clears the previous section of toe. The connecting ligament will then pull the toe back into place almost automatically. This reduces the dislocation. The toe then needs to be buddy taped to the toe or toes next to it for stabilization. A small piece of gauze, cotton, or tissue between the taped toes will prevent skin breakdown if the tape is on for any great length of time. A firm-soled shoe will help keep the toe in line and the foot-toe joint stable. If you are able, ice the toe before buddy taping. Frequent icing and elevation in the next 48 hours is recommended.

To temporarily correct and stabilize an ankle dislocation and related fracture, an orthopedic trauma surgeon recommends straightening the foot by exerting traction in a straight and steady motion—so that as much as possible it is in its natural position and angle to the lower leg. The foot, ankle, and lower leg then need to be stabilized with a splint. Use any available materials to keep the extremity stable. Check the toes frequently for normal skin color and warmth, which indicates good circulation. A dislocated ankle needs to be treated by an emergency room physician or orthopedic surgeon as soon as possible.

If either a toe or ankle dislocation is an "open" dislocation, where the bone has come through the skin, extra care must be taken. This open, or complex, dislocation is usually associated with a fracture, and the bone may still be outside of the skin or may have pulled back inside. First, clean the wound, and then proceed with the reduction. Then, leaving the wound open, apply a sterile dressing, and splint the extremity. Check the end(s) of the extremity farthest from the body to be sure there is adequate circulation, adjusting the extremity as necessary. When the open dislocation is stabilized, seek out immediate medical attention.

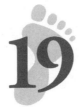

Tendon & Ligament Injuries

The primary function of tendons is to transmit muscle force to the moving joints with limited elongation. Tendons are ropelike structures that attach muscles to bones. Ligaments are similar structures that attach bones to other bones. When muscles and bones move, they exert stresses on the tendons and ligaments that are attached to them. The foot is a complicated but amazing engineering marvel. With 26 bones, 33 joints, 107 ligaments, 19 muscles, and tendons to hold the structure together and allow it to move in a variety of ways, it offers all kinds of opportunities for tendon and ligament injuries.

Troy Marsh, an orthopedic physical therapist, describes tendon disorders as "a major problem among competitive athletes, often interfering with training and competition. Tissue damage may result from a sudden traumatic episode like an ankle sprain, or it may arise with no apparent cause but usually due to cumulative trauma or overuse."

The terms *tendinitis, tendinosis,* and *tendinopathy* all refer to tendon injuries. These terms are commonly confused and misused:

TENDINITIS—The suffix "itis" means inflammation. The term tendinitis should be reserved for tendon injuries that involve larger-scale acute injuries accompanied by inflammation. (Tendinitis is often misspelled as tendonitis, but the preferred spelling used in most of the medical literature is tendinitis.)

TENDINOSIS—The suffix "osis" implies a pathology of chronic degeneration without inflammation. Tendinosis is an accumulation over time of small-scale injuries that don't heal properly; it is a chronic injury of failed healing.

When our muscles move in new ways or do more work than they can easily handle, our muscles and tendons can sustain damage. If the increase in demand is made gradually, muscle and tendon tissues will usually heal, build in strength, and adapt to new loads. It is this principle we use to build muscle and tendon strength.

Many athletes, however, participate in activities that injure a tendon on a microscopic scale and then do more injury before the tendon heals. If you continue the injurious activity, you will gradually accumulate these microinjuries. When enough injury accumulates, you'll feel pain. This kind of injury that comes on slowly with time and persists is a chronic injury; acute tendon injuries are sudden tears that cause immediate pain and obvious symptoms. Tendon injuries often require patience and careful rehabilitation because tendons heal more slowly than muscles.

Tendons are critical for converting the movement of muscle contraction to movement of the foot and/or ankle. The most common tendon injury is to the Achilles tendon, which connects the muscle of the posterior calf to the bottom of the calcaneus bone and mediates plantar flexion (toes down) function across the ankle. Injuries to other tendons that cross the ankle are usually the result of lacerations or direct trauma. Injuries to tendons can vary from mild (stretching) to moderate (tearing) to severe (rupture).

A common tendon problem affects the ankle flexors. These tendons are caught under the pressure of the shoe's tongue and laces across the front top of the foot. Walking or running steep hills can also cause this problem. Another common tendon injury is post-tibial tendinitis. This affects the posterior tibial tendon from the inside of the ankle and the foot. Major tendons and ligaments in the foot and ankle include the following:

- Achilles tendon
- Anterior tibial tendon
- Calcaneofibular ligament

- Inferior talofibular ligament
- Lisfranc ligament
- Peroneal tendons
- Posterior talofibular ligament
- Sinus tarsi syndrome
- Tarsal canal ligaments

Treating Tendon Injuries

There are multiple treatments for tendon injuries. Your podiatrist, sports podiatrist, or orthopedist is the best person to determine the treatment you need. In addition to the treatments below, sometimes a biomechanical assessment is needed. The list below is taken from **Tendinitis.org**, a Website devoted to tendon injuries (the following suggestions for tendinosis also work for tendinitis).

REST. By the time you feel pain from tendinosis, your injury has been gradually building for many weeks. Remember that tendons heal slowly.

PHYSICAL THERAPY EXERCISES can help heal tendinosis, as long as you are careful to progress gradually. Studies have shown that loading a tendon parallel to its length helps the collagen fibers grow with better parallel alignment and speeds the healing process. Find a physical therapist who has a lot of experience with tendinosis, and make sure he/she is willing to go as slowly as your body requires.

SONOCUR SHOCKWAVE THERAPY is a new treatment for tendinosis. The Sonocur machine is an "extracorporeal ultrasound device" that delivers sound waves to a very focused area of the tendon.

ICE is a common treatment for tendinosis. Many physical therapists suggest that you use ice following your exercises or whenever you need some pain reduction during the day. Don't use it just prior to your exercises. It's hard to say if ice has any long-term beneficial effect on tendinosis, but it can be an excellent form of pain control that has no negative side effects (as long as you take care not to get "ice burn" from too much ice).

SUPPORTS AND ORTHOTICS are often used for ankle injuries. Some people find that supports can add stability and support during activity. These should not be worn all the time because you can lose strength and flexibility.

NUTRITIONAL SUPPLEMENTS are somewhat of an unknown area. There has been little scientific research to investigate the effects of nutritional supplements on the healing of tendinosis. Glucosamine sulfate and chondroitin sulfate are not likely to help tendinosis. Other supplements that claim to help heal tendons and ligaments contain the amino acids glycine, lysine, and proline.

BODYWORK is done by physical therapists. Massage and other techniques can help them loosen up and feel better. Many practitioners try to help you with your posture and body mechanics, and some do hands-on soft tissue work.

SURGERY should be a last resort for tendinosis. Some athletes have a positive outcome, while others a negative outcome. Educate yourself about the surgical procedure before you consider it for yourself, and give your injury plenty of time to heal on its own before you resort to surgery.

Troy Marsh reports that "chronic Achilles tendinosis sufferers, most often seen among male recreational runners between 35 and 45 years old, responded favorably to a 12-week training program of high-load eccentric calf muscle training and returned to full running activity. A comparison group with the same diagnosis, treated conventionally with anti-inflammatory drugs, orthotics, rest, and therapy modalities, was not successful and each subject ultimately was treated surgically."

How Tendons Heal

Tendons have limited blood supply and nutrition is often supported via synovial fluid within the presence of a tendon sheath. In other words, tendons are designed to transmit tensile loads, have limited elastic properties, and heal slowly compared to other more oxygenated tissue. This is important to know as one begins to understand the basis of optimal healing after injury and repair. It is very important to understand if prevention and performance is in mind.

Optimal healing consists of three phases, namely, inflammation, repair, and remodeling. The first three days after acute tendon injury sees inflammation. During this time tendons are most sensitive to mechanical load and are chemically irritated. Relative rest is indicated. Interestingly, after about three weeks, inflammatory cells are not present and medications may lose the desired effect.

Repair of damaged tissue lasts about four to six weeks and consists of the deposition of new collagen. Early mobilization is a key factor for strengthening the repairing tendon and begins the process of organizing the new collagen along the lines of functional stress. Prolonged rest may not provide the controlled loading stimulus necessary for maturation of the healing tissue and may actually set up a degenerative process—a condition referred to as tendinosis.

Remodeling is the process of reorganizing the "contracted and disorganized" collagen fibers. Effective remodeling requires a progressive return to normal loads and activity to prevent contractures and to promote strength and flexibility. This process may take up to a year to mature and should include all three planes of functional motion. The three planes of motion at the foot and ankle can be appreciated when running trails as the surface becomes uneven or pitched, or when sharp turn angles are required.

Targeting tendon tissue for early treatment should focus on aerobic training and has been shown to increase tensile strength and endurance. This means high repetitions (100 to 200 per set) with low loads and introducing eccentric loading as soon as tolerable. Eccentric loading, unlike its concentric counterpart, is the lengthening of muscle under load. For example, a single leg heel raise using one's own body weight is concentric on the up phase and eccentric on the down phase. Standing toe raises are effective in strengthening tendons on the front of the ankle.

—Troy Marsh, an orthopedic physical therapist

Marsh suggests "remembering to keep the proximal muscle groups such as the hips and thighs strong and responsive in all planes of motion. Integrating functional and sport-specific strength and balance exercises, such as single leg heel raises, into your training will enhance performance, and hopefully, prevent any serious tendon disorders—and prepare you for the next athletic event."

Further information including reports on medical studies can be found at **www.tendinosis.org/index.html.**

Achilles Tendinitis

The Achilles tendon connects the gastrocnemius and the soleus, the two major muscles of the calf, to the heel bone. It stabilizes the heel every time you take a step. The tendon makes it possible for you to rise up on your toes, run, and jump. Achilles tendinitis occurs when the sheath surrounding this cord becomes inflamed. There may be small tears in the tendon, or sudden and repeated stretching of the tendon causes an inflammation that is painful behind the heel, ankle, and lower calf while walking and running. The pain may be felt during the early part of your run or hike, and then subside, only to worsen after stopping. This pain is your first warning, followed by swelling of the Achilles tendon, and pain to touch at the base of your heel.

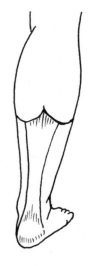

The Achilles tendon

A mild first-degree injury makes it difficult to rise up on your toes or walk on your heels. With proper treatment, you should be able to walk with little pain after about 48 hours. You should not resume normal athletic activity for several weeks. A second-degree injury is when there is partial tearing of the tendon from its attachment point. This injury will take from six to eight weeks to heal, with an additional two to four weeks of stretching exercises before normal athletic activity can be resumed. In a third-degree injury, an extreme case, the Achilles tendon ruptures. This requires immediate medical intervention, usually surgery, and a long healing and strengthening process. There is sudden calf pain and usually an audible snap if the tendon ruptures. The tendon will ball up in the calf with a related defect in the lower tendon. If the tendon is swollen, or you suspect a tear, usually a second- or third-degree injury, you should not risk running on it. You can further damage or rupture the tendon. If the pain is mild and goes away in five minutes with a warm-up, typically a first-degree injury, it is usually OK to continue.

A sudden increase in activity, increasing your mileage too fast, or running steep hills can lead to an inflamed Achilles tendon. To prevent Achilles tendon problems, increase your activity, mileage, and hill training gradually. Proper lower leg muscle stretching can also help prevent problems. Overpronators, whose arch collapses when walking or running, are more prone than others to Achilles problems.

Rich Schick, a physician's assistant, adds the following:

> The Achilles tendon is not a simple structure. It is more correctly termed the Achilles complex. If it were as simple as we perceive it, there would be a straight pull from the calf muscle to the heel and the tendon would be very prominent instead of following the contour of the leg. In reality the tendon passes through a series of little tunnels of very tough tissue that hold it close to the leg.
>
> In severe cases of Achilles tendinitis, calcium deposits can form in and on the tendon, preventing it from passing through these little tunnels and resulting in a permanent disability or the need for surgery. This is called calcific tendinitis. If you grasp the tendon between your thumb and forefinger, move your foot up and down, and feel a grating or bubble-popping sensation, this is a sign of serious tendinitis. The finding is called *crepitus* and represents severe inflammation. If not treated appropriately, it can lead to calcific tendinitis. You must stop using the leg as much as possible. Some authorities recommend casting until this goes away. Ice and anti-inflammatory medication are also helpful.

Ignoring the signs of Achilles tendinitis and not seeking treatment can lead to a chronic inflammation or even tendon rupture. The pain may occur when warming up and then ease up. The athlete continues to train and the pain returns after the session has ended. Over time, the periods of pain-free training become shorter and shorter. Eventually, training may become impossible and treatment mandatory. This can lead to formation of a cyst in the tendon. As the cyst expands, the tendon thins out and becomes more susceptible to rupture if overstressed.

Treating Achilles Tendinitis

The major causes of Achilles tendon problems are a lack of strength and flexibility in the calf muscles, a weakness in the tendon, or a weak ankle joint. Treatment may include any or all of the following: icing as described below, stretching and flexibility exercises, wearing flexible shoes or boots with a well-padded heel counter, and avoiding the ups and downs of hills.

If you suspect you have Achilles tendinitis, stop running—do not run through the pain. Ignoring the symptoms may cause the tendon to rupture, which usually requires surgery. Call your orthopedist or podiatrist if the pain persists. The doctor may put your foot in either a flexible or immobilizing cast to reduce movement and weight bearing. Once the cast is removed, you will need to do stretching exercises to strengthen the tendon before resuming normal athletic activity.

The treatment for a mildly injured Achilles tendinitis is the same RICE treatment used for ankle sprains and strains: rest, ice, compression, and elevation. The first 24 hours are the most critical for beginning treatment. Early treatment decreases swelling and lessens the risk of additional injury. Initial rest of the foot is also important. A lightly wound Ace wrap will provide compression to help keep swelling down while providing support. Apply the Ace wrap from the forefoot upwards towards the calf. Do not wear the Ace wrap to bed at night. Apply ice for 20 minutes at a time three to four times daily. Ice can be very helpful in the healing process. Refer to the chapter "Cold & Heat Therapy" for more information on making the most of icing techniques. See also "Supplements for Quick Recovery" on page 234.

The injured area should be elevated above the level of the heart as much as possible during the first 48 hours. This keeps blood away from the injured area and reduces pain and swelling. The use of anti-inflammatory medications is usually warranted.

A small heel pad will alleviate the stresses on the tendon. For some individuals, wearing low-heeled shoes as often as possible will help keep the

Achilles tendon stretched. An Achilles notch in shoes or mid- and low-top boots will accommodate the Achilles tendon in plantar flexion. The Achilles Tendon Strap made by Cho-Pat can provide relief from the discomfort of Achilles tendinitis.

A lightweight plastic night splint worn to bed can help to stretch the foot, limit contraction of soft tissues at night, and avoid morning stiffness. Night splints help avoid footdrop and accompanying muscle tightening. Night splints are proven as a treatment method for preventing the plantar fascia and Achilles tendon from contracting during the night. Many athletes swear by them. Check with your podiatrist, orthopedist, or medical supply store. Several night splint models are available. If the pain persists, consult a medical specialist. He or she will need to rule out partial tears of the tendon, an inflammation of the tendon's sheath, or degenerative changes.

Rupture of the tendon requires specialized care. If the rupture is fresh, within hours of the injury, surgical repair of the tendon is usually done. Older injuries may also be treated surgically, though many patients will improve by casting the leg. Diminished strength and rerupture is more frequently seen in patients who are casted without surgery, so preference is to surgically repair the rupture. Following surgical repair of Achilles tendon injuries, the patient is usually casted; then when the cast is removed, the patient receives extensive rehabilitation to regain strength and flexibility. Often a heel lift is required for from six months to a year after the cast has been removed.

Exercises to Stretch the Achilles Tendon

Stretching helps athletes improve flexibility and counter muscular imbalances that put them at a greater risk of injury. Proper stretching of the Achilles tendon can help prevent an Achilles injury.

One method of stretching is to stand far enough from a wall or heavy piece of furniture so that when you lean forward towards the wall or furniture you can feel the tendons stretch in the back of your leg while keeping your feet flat on the floor. Lean forward and stretch only to the point of feeling the stretch, not to the point of feeling pain. Alternate a 20 seconds stretch with a 20 second rest standing straight; repeat 10 to 20 times. Continue this daily stretching until the Achilles stops hurting.

Dr. Les Appel, who designed the Powerstep Insole, recommends facing a wall with one foot flat on the floor and the other foot's heel on the floor and toes up on the wall 3 to 4 inches. Gently move your knee slowly towards the wall until you feel slight stretching on the bottom of your foot and the back of your leg. Hold this position for 30 seconds, and repeat five times per foot.

A Swedish study showed excellent results with a simple stretch. Stand on a step or ledge on the balls of your feet. Push yourself up with your good leg and slowly transfer your weight to the affected leg. Slowly lower yourself all the way down until the injured leg's heel is below the stair level and you feel the pull on the soleus calf muscle. Alternate this stretch with the injured leg's knee straight and then slightly bent. Repeat three sets of 15, twice a day. Additional strength can be gained by adding weight over time. Use dumbbells, a light barbell, or a weighted backpack.

The ProStretch is a popular tool to effectively stretch the plantar fascia as well as the Achilles tendon and the gastrocnemius and soleus musculature of the back of the lower leg. Studies have shown that utilization of the ProStretch can more effectively increase ankle dorsiflexion (toe-up motion of the ankle) than the conventional and commonly used wall stretch technique mentioned above.[26] Its use is recommended as both a preventive measure and a treatment technique.

ACHILLES-TENDINITIS PRODUCTS

The **ACHILLES HEALER** reduces stress on the Achilles tendon. The strap is made from ProWrap, a knitted blend of nylon and Lycra with patented foam lining. **Fabrifoam Products, (800) 577-1077, www.fabrifoam.com**

The **ACHILLOTRAIN** is a lightweight, breathable sock that offers support for the Achilles tendon. It has silicone inserts in the back of the heel and under it. **Bauerfeind USA, Inc., (800) 423-3405, www.bauerfeindusa.com**

CHO-PAT'S ACHILLES TENDON STRAP fits under the arch and around the ankle to relieve pressure on the Achilles tendon. Trials at the Mayo's Sports/ Medicine Clinic have shown the strap effective as an addition to traditional treatments for Achilles tendinitis, particularly during the push-off phase of gait. The strap is available in four sizes based on ankle circumference at its widest point. **Cho-Pat, Inc., (800) 221-1601, www.cho-pat.com**

ACHILLES-TENDINITIS PRODUCTS

ENGO PERFORMANCE PATCHES are made of a thin fabric-film composite that can greatly reduce friction in targeted locations within your footwear. The patches can give a slick, slippery surface to the heel counter of your footwear or insole where Achilles tendon friction is a problem. Patches come in three sizes: small ovals, large ovals, and sheets, and they can be trimmed for a custom fit. Each patch is extremely durable, lasting anywhere from several weeks to several months. **Tamarack Habilitation Technologies Inc., (763) 795-0057, www.goengo.com**

HAPAD THREE-QUARTER-LENGTH HEEL WEDGES provide the necessary heel lift to help reduce the pain associated with Achilles tendinitis. They are available in three thicknesses. The coiled, springlike wool fibers provide firm and resilient support as they mold and shape to the foot. **Hapad, (800) 544-2723, www.hapad.com**

The **N'ICE STRETCH NIGHT SPLINT SUSPENSION SYSTEM** is made for both Achilles tendinitis and plantar fasciitis. This night splint uses bilateral suspension straps to provide continuous nighttime stretching of the Achilles tendon and plantar fasciitis. The straps allow for independent bi-plane dorsiflexion adjustment. A removable Sealed Ice pack provides cold therapy coupled with stretching of soft tissues. The unit is hinged to fold compactly. **Brown Medical Industries, (800) 843-4395, www.brownmed.com**

The **PROSTRETCH** is a popular tool that effectively stretches the Achilles tendon, the plantar fascia, and the calf muscles. It builds lower extremity strength, balance, and flexibility benefits in three minutes of use prior to activity, thus reducing the risk of injury. The PT100 is unilateral, the PT200 bilateral. Both models can also be used for hamstring and anterior tibialis stretching. **ProStretch at Prism Enterprises, (800) 535-3629, www.prostretch.com**

The **TP MASSAGE FOOTBALLER** was created to relieve plantar fasciitis, Achilles tendinitis, and heel pain. It works on the muscle of existing "spasms" and/or "trigger points" by applying pressure to the "trigger point" area. **Trigger Point Technologies, (888) 312-2557, www .tpmassageball.com**

Bursitis

Bursa are small fluid-filled sacs found between areas of high friction such as where muscles or tendons glide over bone. The bursa acts as a shock absorber, allowing movement between neighboring structures, usually in opposite directions. The body has more than 150 bursa sacs. Bursitis is the formation of an inflamed fluid-filled sac from trauma or overuse. On the feet, bursitis may develop beneath a callus or a bunion, under the metatarsal heads, or at the heel.

Typical causes of bursitis in the feet can be repetitive motions or an injury or sustained pressure to a joint. As the usually slippery bursa sac becomes inflamed, it loses it gliding capabilities and becomes gritty and rough. Inflamed bursas are painful and irritating. Bursitis in the heel can manifest itself with the same symptoms as plantar fasciitis, but the heel bursitis will persist with any weight-bearing activity, whereas with plantar fasciitis the symptoms are relieved after the fascia warms up.

Treating Bursitis

The first action is to stop or reduce the motion or action that is causing the bursitis. The use of NSAIDS will help reduce the inflammation. Heat will relax the joint and promote tissue repair. In severe cases, fluid may be drawn from the sac to relieve pressure. Gently warming up before strenuous exercise can help avoid bursitis. If you experience chronic bursitis, ask your doctor about medications and treatment options to relieve the pain and discomfort.

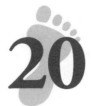

Heel Problems

The heel bone, called the *calcaneus,* is the largest bone in the foot and absorbs most of the shock and pressure from walking and running. The most common cause of heel pain is incorrect movement of the foot during running, hiking, or walking. With every heel strike, pressure up to four times the body's weight is placed on the heel, flattening the heel's fat pads and sending shock and stress to the bones of the foot and the arch. Some of the shock and stress travels on up the leg. As we age, the thickness of the heel's fat pads and the fat pads under the balls of our feet decreases; our natural shock absorption is reduced, pressure is increased, and we become more susceptible to injury. Heel pain may be caused by heel-pain syndrome, heel spurs, plantar fasciitis, or Haglund's deformity.

Heel pain can also be caused by dry and cracked skin at the back and bottom of the heel. This skin is often built up into a callus, and the fissures in the skin can be painful. Treat this problem the same as any callus (see page 297).

Heel-Pain Syndrome

Heel-pain syndrome is usually caused by overuse of and repetitive stress on the foot's heel. This can be caused by a sudden increase in athletic activity, shoes with heels that are too low or that have lost their cushioning, or by the thinning of the fat pad on the bottom of the heels. This can be resolved by increasing our activity level slowly, by wearing shoes with good cushioning, or by using a heel pad or cup.

Heel Spurs & Plantar Fasciitis

Heel pain may also be caused by heel spurs or plantar fasciitis, which arise from the heel bone and attached soft tissues being stressed. This type of heel pain is often the worst in the morning after getting out of bed and putting your feet on the floor—sometimes it improves after a few minutes. The section on plantar fasciitis (see below) should be considered mandatory reading for any athlete experiencing heel pain. Heel spurs and plantar fasciitis are closely related, and those with heel pain can benefit from many of the same treatments, stretches, and products.

Heel Spurs

Heel spurs are small points of calcium buildup sticking out and downward from the "calcaneus" heel bone, touching and irritating your plantar fascia. (Painful protrusions on the back of the heel are called Haglund's deformity; see page 270.) Stresses to the plantar fascia where it inserts into the calcaneus causes heel spurs to develop. A heel spur can usually be seen on an X-ray. A heel bruise or stone bruise is pain felt directly under the calcaneus. This pain is usually tenderness at a small site just forward of the heel's pad on the bottom of the heel.

Achilles tendinitis, flat feet, and excessively high arches are common conditions that make one prone to heel spurs.

Treating Heel Spurs

Proper conditioning of the feet and gradually working up to longer distances can help minimize heel pain. Many stretches can help prevent and also treat heel spurs, as well as plantar fasciitis (see section on stretching below).

Resting your feet and using ice is helpful when you first experience pain—ice 20 minutes three to four times a day for several days. The "Cold & Heat Therapy" chapter gives more information on making the most of icing techniques. As pain subsides over time, warm soaks can help.

Tom Noll found his solution to heel pain by experimenting with different running shoes and the use of arch supports. By participating in discussions on a Web-based email listserv, Noll began to see similarities as some people mentioned that they too had problems with the same model shoe he was wearing. He changed shoes and determined that he needed the arch support in all his shoes.

One very basic but important recommendation is to never walk in bare feet until you are pain free—especially in the morning getting out of bed. Keep a pair of shoes with an arch support at your bedside. Use sandals only if they have an arch support.

The use of orthotics in resolving heel pain has been proven. The biggest issue with custom orthotics is their cost. Many athletes first try an inexpensive over-the-counter orthotic. If that does not work, the more expensive custom-made orthotic may be necessary (see the "Orthotics" chapter, page 121, for detailed information on common types of orthotics).

The products listed below are quite varied. Some heel cups have a waffle design or special-density bottom material on the bottom of the cup; others have a U-shape cutout at the bottom of the heel. Most heel cups simply cup the heel, while others are incorporated into a sock design. The new viscoelastic materials in some heel pads provide excellent cushioning. Heel pads are small and fit easily into a shoe to provide cushioning. Try several to find a design that works best for your pain or injury. Heel cups and pads are small and can easily be carried as preventive measures if you are prone to heel pain. The Count'R-Force Arch Brace and the PSC strap are alternatives to heel cups and pads.

Plantar Fasciitis

The plantar fascia is a band of connective fibrous tissue that runs from the heel to the ball of the foot, forming the foot's arch. The band helps in support and stabilization of the foot during hiking and running. The arch flattens when standing. As you begin a step the heel lifts up and also the plantar fascia tightens to form the curve of the arch and provides a strong push off with the toes. An inflammation of the fascia, called *plantar fasciitis,* occurs most often with overuse. The stretching and tearing of some of the fibers in the plantar fascia as it inserts into the heel bone causes the inflammation. If you have flat feet or high arches, or if you overpronate, the plantar fascia is strained, mainly at the heel. The stresses of impact sports, running, and hiking may flatten, lengthen, and eventually cause small tears in the plantar fascia. Tears near the heel bone often cause a heel spur to develop.

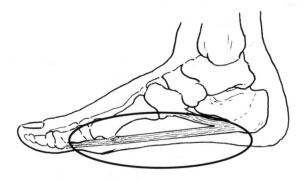

The plantar fascia.

Athletes who are predisposed to plantar fasciitis injuries typically have increased their mileage too fast, increased the frequency and intensity of their workouts, increased the amount of hill work, and/or have a lack of flexibility and strength in their ankle and foot. They may also have a foot imbalance such as flat feet or high arches.

Plantar fascia pain is commonly felt in the morning or after long periods of sitting. The first steps at these times cause a sudden strain to the band of tissue that has started to heal itself during the night. The pain and stiffness is usually centered at the bottom of the heel, but symptoms may radiate into the arch. Although the pain may decrease somewhat with your initial activity, as the day progresses, it may return and be quite painful.

Consult your podiatrist or orthopedist if you are suffering from pain in the arch of your foot or suspect that you have plantar fasciitis. An aggressive multidisciplined medical approach using medical, biomechanical, and physical therapy treatments can help to return you to action as soon as possible. The Achilles tendon may also be involved, causing pain under the foot as it stretches.

Treating Plantar Fasciitis

Generally prescribed treatments for plantar fasciitis include rest, moist heat and stretching in the morning or before activity, icing massage after activity, using heel cups, changing insoles or adding an arch support, taping of the foot or an arch brace, orthotics, foot exercises, and shoe modifications. Ice your heels and the bottom of your foot after exercise (see the chapter "Cold & Heat Therapy" for information on making the most of icing techniques). By all means, replace your worn out shoes and insoles. Usually you need either to provide more support to the arch or lessen the amount of overpronation. An arch support or arch pad can provide pain relief. Motion-control shoes can help if you overpronate. In extreme cases, oral anti-inflammatory medications, cortisone injections, physical therapy, cast immobilization, and even surgery may be necessary.

The first thing any doctor or physical therapist should tell you is to stop all impact activities for a period of weeks or months and to always wear shoes. Going barefoot is one of the worst things someone suffering from plantar fasciitis can do. Keep in mind that the tiny tears need to heal, and it makes sense to stop the activity that caused them in the first place. Have shoes by your bedside in case you have to get up at night. Avoid sandals unless they have an arch support.

You also need to regain flexibility and elasticity in the soleus muscle/sheath to prevent the condition from occurring again. Stretching is the way to do that, but you have to start out slow and easy, that is, writing the alphabet with your foot in warm bath water. (See the section on stretching below for various useful exercises for increasing flexibility.) Once you've started to heal, you can move on to the more demanding stretches. The most common comment by those who have conquered plantar fasciitis is how stretching helped more than anything else. A physical therapist or chiropractor can help adjust muscle imbalances.

A study by the American Orthopaedic Foot and Ankle Society looked at heel pain related to plantar fasciitis.[26] Dr. Glenn Pfeffer reported chronic heel pain as the most common foot problem, with up to 80 percent caused by proximal plantar fasciitis. The study compared a common polypropylene custom orthotic device, three over-the-counter heel pads (a Viscoheel silicone heel cushion, a Tuli's Heel Cup, and a Hapad Comforthotic), and stretching alone. After comparing the results of five control groups, they found that stretching and off-the-shelf shoe inserts were just as effective as stretching and the more costly orthotics. Their recommendation: "For the initial treatment of heel pain, stretching, and a simple, inexpensive, off-the-shelf device is the best way to go." When wearing heel pads, be sure to use them in all your shoes.

In an interesting article, "Plantar Fasciitis—A New Perspective,"[27] Robert Nirschl, MD, makes a case for plantar fasciitis as a painful degenerative plantar tendinitis, not an inflammation problem. His research found no inflammatory cells in injured plantar fascia—meaning that anti-inflammatory medications and cortisone will not have curative potential. For plantar tendinitis Dr. Nirschl recommends stretching and strength training all areas of the leg to restore strength, endurance, and flexibility. Also recommended is the use of a night splint, arch bracing or a soft orthotic, and footwear with good midfoot flexibility. In extreme cases, surgery may be indicated to remove painful tendinitis tissue. If your plantar fascia pain does not respond to prescribed treatment, consider asking your podiatrist or orthopedist to look into this study.

Orthotics will often help relieve plantar-fascia pain. AliMed Rehab and Apex make orthotics for plantar fasciitis. Gary Buffington recommends trying inexpensive orthotic shoe inserts before you have expensive orthotics made. Gary suggests you "wear them always until you are better—even in your bedroom slippers if you go to the bathroom at night. I think it would be best if you never took a step without them under your foot for a month. Also two Aleve tablets twice a day; and contrast baths of two buckets of water, one at 68 degrees, the other 103 degrees. Five minutes in hot, two in cold, five in hot, two in cold, and then five more in the hot for a total of 19 minutes twice a day or more." Following that regimen for one year got Gary through the Boston Marathon.

It is possible to tape the plantar fascia area under the foot for support, though doing so can be hard to manage. The tape, however, loses strength as it moves with the skin—40 percent of its strength can be lost within 20 minutes. Using one of the supports listed below will work better over time. An arch brace wraps around the arch to provide support and decrease the pull of the plantar fascia on the calcaneus heel bone. The Count'R-Force Arch Brace and the PSC wrap are two wraparound supports that provide relief from plantar-fasciitis pain. The Hapad Longitudinal Metatarsal Arch Pads or 3-Way Heel/Arch/Metatarsal Insoles may also be used to relieve pain.

Lightweight plastic night splints are proven as a treatment for preventing the plantar fascia and Achilles tendon from contracting during the night. Many athletes swear by them. The splint helps stretch the foot, limit contraction of soft tissues at night, and avoid morning stiffness. Night splints also help avoid footdrop and accompanying muscle tightening. Check with your podiatrist, orthopedist, or medical supply store. Several night splint models are available. The Strassburg Sock is an alternative-style night splint that can be worn at night or while resting to lightly stretch the plantar fascia.

If the problem persists after trying some of these measures, make an appointment with a podiatrist or orthopedist. Advances in medical technology have resulted in the use of shock waves to reduce the troublesome inflammation and help jumpstart blood flow that in turn reduces pain and encourages healing. Common sense should tell you to try other conservative treatments before moving to the shock-wave treatment or surgery.

Orthotripsy (shock-wave therapy) uses high-energy shock waves similar to those used for treating kidney stones. Shock-wave therapy is indicated for the use with patients suffering from chronic plantar fasciitis and heel-pain syndrome who fail to respond to the traditional and conservative treatments. The procedure is noninvasive. Check with your podiatrist to find a specialist in your area who is trained in this new technology.

Endoscopic plantar fasciotomy is an invasive procedure in which a specialized camera is inserted into the heel area. Using the camera, the surgeon can see the plantar fascia through a very small incision, less than ½ inch, and release the extreme tension on the plantar fascia.

Stretching Exercises for Heel Spurs & Plantar Fasciitis

Athletes can improve their flexibility and counter muscular imbalances that put them at a greater risk of injury by following a simple stretching program. The best results may come from a combination of plantar fascia and Achilles tendon stretching in multiple directions.

Morning Stretches

- Before getting out of bed, lie on your stomach, put your toes and forefoot against the mattress, and straighten your leg so your heel stretches your calf muscle. This can make your first steps less painful.

- Also before getting out of bed, slowly stretch the toes upward towards the head at least three times per day, holding the stretch for at least 15 seconds.

- Stretch the Achilles tendon by bending the knee with the ankle flexed back towards you and gently pulling your toes back towards your knee. Hold this pull to a count of 10 and repeat 6 to 10 times a day. Using a towel around your toes to pull them towards you is an alternative.

- Another effective morning calf stretch is to stand facing a wall with your hands on the wall. Extend one foot behind you about 24 inches, while bending the other leg at the knee. Keep the heel of the back foot flat on the floor for two minutes and keep the knee straight—you will feel the calf muscle stretch. Repeat with the other foot.

Other Effective Stretches

- Dr. Pam Adams suggests toe curls to strengthen your arch to prevent pronation. Sit down, take your shoes off, and curl your toes under as hard as you can and as many times as you can. In the beginning, you might get a cramp. Just walk around and try the curls again. Dr. Adams is a chiropractor who offers Painless Guides at **www.painlessguides.com.**

- An easy and effective exercise is to sit on a stool or other surface that permits your legs to dangle and point your toes downward as you draw the alphabet in the air. Repeat three to five times.

- Dr. Les Appel, who designed the Powerstep Insole, recommends facing a wall with one foot flat on the floor and the other foot's heel on the floor and toes up on the wall 3 to 4 inches. Gently move your knee slowly towards the wall until you feel slight stretching on the bottom of your foot and the back of your leg. Curl your toes to raise the arch and transfer your weight to the outside of your foot. Uncurl your toes, hold for 30 seconds, and again curl your toes. Hold each position for 30 seconds, repeating five times per position per foot.

- Rolling a tennis ball back and forth under the arch of the foot or simple self-massage across and along the arch can also help. Ice massage can be done using a small frozen juice rolled under your arch.

- Stand balancing on the foot with plantar fasciitis symptoms whenever possible.

- Better than a tennis ball is the TP Massage FootBaller. Apply pressure with the FootBaller by using the floor, a table, or any hard surface to allow slight movement of your foot on the device. As pressure is applied, the material will slightly change shape in about 5 to 7 seconds. As the materials change shape, roll the footballer to and fro covering the entire affected area of the foot so that the "trigger point" or "spasm" is relieved.

- The ProStretch is a popular tool to effectively stretch the plantar fascia as well as the Achilles tendon and the gastrocnemius and soleus musculature of the back of the lower leg. Studies have shown that utilization of the ProStretch can more effectively increase ankle dorsiflexion (toe-up motion of the ankle) than the conventional and commonly used wall stretch technique mentioned above.[28] Its use is recommended as both a preventive measure as well as a treatment technique.

HEEL SPURS & PLANTAR FASCIITIS

ACCOMMODATOR ORTHOTICS provide relief from heel pain and plantar fasciitis. The High-Impact Accommodator offers the benefit of an Impact Plus energy-absorbing poromeric polymer pad in the heel. The Viscoelastic Accommodator combines Accommodator and three-quarter–length design with the proven attributes of a pure, supple, viscoelastic polymer. Each offers a shaped longitudinal arch to relieve fatigue while supporting the arch, and a mild metatarsal arch, which supports and reduces unnecessary pressure from the metatarsal heads. **AliMed Inc., (800) 225-2610, www.alimed.com**

The **COUNT'R-FORCE ARCH BRACE**, an alternative to taping, is ideal for running and hiking. Designed by Robert Nirschi, MD, an orthopedic surgeon/sports medicine specialist, it has a curved shape that allow a wide distribution of the abusive forces causing the heel and plantar-fasciitis pain. Two tension straps allow for personal adjustment. **Medical Sports, Inc., (800) 783-2240, www.medsports.com**

CRAMER HEEL CUPS offer a basic heel cup that is made with Provosane II bonded to a layer of soft polyurethane foam. **Cramer Products Inc. (800) 255-6621, www.cramersportsmed.com**

HAPAD ARCH PADS can relieve the discomfort of plantar fasciitis. The Longitudinal Metatarsal Arch Pads provide a corrective action that strengthens the longitudinal and metatarsal arches without restricting the natural flexibility of the foot. These pads may also help flat feet. The 3-Way Heel/Arch/Metatarsal Insoles is an all-in-one Longitudinal Metatarsal Arch Cushion and heel cushion that relieves plantar fasciitis and foot fatigue by supporting the arch, cushioning the heel, and distributing pressure across the ball of the foot. The Comf-Orthotic Three-Quarter–Length Insole is a contoured one-piece arch, metatarsal, and heel cushion that helps support flat feet. **Hapad, (800) 544-2723, www.hapad.com**

HAPAD HEEL PADS AND CUSHIONS are useful in treating heel pain associated with stone bruises, heel spurs, leg-length discrepancies, and Achilles tendinitis. The Horseshoe Heel Pads relieve heel pain, and the Medial/Lateral Heel Wedges helps correct misalignment of the heel and ankle. The Comf-Orthotic Three-Quarter–Length Insole is a contoured one-piece arch,

HEEL SPURS & PLANTAR FASCIITIS

metatarsal, and heel cushion that relieves heel spur pain. The coiled, spring-like wool fibers provide firm and resilient support as they mold and shape to the foot. **Hapad, (800) 544-2723, www.hapad.com**

The **HEEL HUGGER** is designed to treat heel pain and inflammatory problems of the heel. The neoprene sock surrounds the foot from the heel to the mid-foot providing support, stabilization, and compression to control edema. Therapeutic Gel pads with Sealed Ice provide additional stabilization and cold therapy on either side of the calcaneus heel bone. The Heel Hugger provides relief from heel spurs, plantar fasciitis, Achilles tendinitis, heel contusions, narrow heels, and rear-foot instability. **Brown Medical Industries, (800) 843-4395, www.brownmed.com**

The **LYNCO BIOMECHANICAL ORTHOTIC SYSTEM** is a "ready-made" triple-density orthotic system that comes in enough variations to accommodate 90 percent of foot disorders, including plantar fasciitis. Each model has either a neutral-cupped heel or a medial posted heel, and comes with or without a metatarsal pad. Additional Reflex self-adhesive pads can be added to the orthotics to relieve pain from Morton's toe, sesamoiditis, and leg-length discrepancy. **APEX Foot Health Industries, (800) 526-APEX, www.apexfoot.com**

The **N'ICE STRETCH NIGHT SPLINT SUSPENSION SYSTEM** is made for plantar fasciitis and Achilles tendinitis. It uses bilateral suspension straps to provide continuous nighttime stretching of the plantar fasciitis and Achilles tendon. The straps allow for independent biplane dorsiflexion adjustment. A removable Sealed Ice pack provides cold therapy. The unit is hinged to fold compactly. **Brown Medical Industries, (800) 843-4395, www.brownmed.com**

The **ORTHO SLIPPER** was designed by Dr. W. E. Nordt, an orthopedic surgeon. This soft slipper is worn as a night splint to relieve the symptoms of heel pain and plantar fasciitis. **Nordt Device, (866) 683-7873, www.dynaslipper.com**

The **PF NIGHT SPLINT** comes in three models to relieve the pain of plantar fasciitis. The Original PF Night Splint is a lightweight plastic splint designed to lessen morning pain caused by contractures and muscle tightening while sleeping. The Freedom PF Night Splint II is a low-profile lighter weight splint,

HEEL SPURS & PLANTAR FASCIITIS

and the Soft PF Night Splint is made for sleeping but allows ambulation. All splints fit both right and left feet and include a liner and straps to protect the leg and instep from pressure. An extra-wide model of the PF Night Splint is offered for those individuals with larger calves and ankles. **AliMed, (800) 225-2610, www.alimed.com**

POWERSTEPS INSOLES by Dr. Les Appel offer a unique four-phase design to relieve heel and arch pain. Made with a strong prescription-like arch support, it has a strong heel cradle that prevents the foot from pronating (rolling inward) and the arch from flattening—eliminating strain on the plantar fascia. **Stable Step, (888) 237-3668, www.powersteps.com**

The **PROSTRETCH** is a popular tool that effectively stretches the plantar fascia, the Achilles tendon, and the calf muscles. It builds lower-extremity strength, balance, and flexibility in three minutes of use prior to activity, thus reducing the risk of injury. The PT100 is unilateral, the PT200 bilateral. Both models can also be used for hamstring and anterior tibialis stretching. **Medi-Dyne, (800) 810-1740, www.medi-dyne.com**

The **PSC–PRONATION/SPRING CONTROL** strap is designed to treat plantar fasciitis, chronic heel pain, heel spur syndrome, and shin splints. This reusable strapping device is made from ProWrap, a knitted blend of nylon and Lycra with patented foam lining. It wraps around the arch to provide superior support to the plantar fascia while also wrapping around the heel to reduce the force of heel strike and biomechanically move the foot's midline to a more neutral position. **Fabrifoam Products, (800) 577-1077, www.fabrifoam.com**

SPENCO CUSHIONS are made from a noncompressible, viscoelastic material to relieve heel pain associated with heel spurs, thinning heel pads, and plantar fasciitis. Products include ViscoSpot and ViscoHeel cushions; Ipos Shock Absorber Heel cushions and SoftBase Insoles; and ViscoPed insoles. They reduce shock to the joints and evenly distribute pressure throughout the cushion. Available at sporting-goods stores and some drugstores.

HEEL SPURS & PLANTAR FASCIITIS

The **STRASSBURG SOCK** is easy to use at night or during extended periods of rest. A good alternative to the typical night splint, this system can be easily used and carried while backpacking. A standard over-the-calf tube sock uses two adjustable straps: one around the calf just below the knee; the other attached to the toe of the sock and passed through a D ring on the upper strap. Tension on the toe strap keeps the plantar fascia in a neutral to slightly stretched position, reducing or eliminating pain under the heel during initial weight bearing in the morning. **JT Enterprises, (800) 452-0631, www.thesock.com**

The **TP MASSAGE FOOTBALLER** was created to relieve plantar fasciitis, Achilles tendinitis, and heel pain. It works on the muscle of existing "spasms" and/or "trigger points" by applying pressure to the "trigger point" area. This unique product has received rave reviews from its users. **Trigger Point Technologies, (888) 312-2557, www.tpmassageball.com**

TULI'S makes different versions of heel cups with a waffle design. The Standard design is single-ribbed, the Pro Heel Cup has a double-ribbed waffle design, and the Gel Heel Cup is double-ribbed with gel polymer. For those with weak ankles, the Cheetah Neoprene Ankle Support incorporates a standard heel cup with a neoprene ankle sock-type support. **Medi-Dyne, (800) 810-1740, www.medi-dyne.com**

The **ULTIMATE HEEL & ARCH SUPPORT**, designed by foot-care specialist Dr. G. Budak, is made from viscoelastic polymer that molds to the foot, forms a deep heel cup, and follows the contour of the arch, thereby making a custom fit. As a three-quarter–length orthotic, it provides relief from plantar fasciitis, heel spur pain, Achilles tendinitis, and arch, knee, and back strain. It also absorbs up to 90 percent of impact shock, which reduces stress to the heel, foot, leg, and back. **(866) 923-9000, www.footwork.net**

VISCOPED S INSOLES are made from a noncompressible viscoelastic material with a bar of softer silicon in the metatarsal and heel areas that is designed to relieve plantar-fascia pain. The insole reduces shock throughout the entire length of the insole and distributes pressure evenly. **Bauerfeind USA, (800) 423-3405, www.bauerfeindusa.com**

Haglund's Deformity

Haglund's deformity is a bump in the form of an enlargement of the back of the heel bone (calcaneus) at the area of the insertion of the Achilles tendon. Sometimes it has the appearance of a square, shelflike bump. When the bump is irritated by the wearing of shoes, it becomes red, swollen, and painful. The enlarged bone may also irritate the Achilles tendon, resulting in pain with motion of the ankle joint and foot. Shoes with a rigid heel counter rub up and down on the heel bone. There is a bursa sac between the Achilles tendon and the heel bone that becomes irritated and over time bursitis may develop.

Haglund's deformity is also called "pump bump" or *retrocalcaneal bursitis.* It may be a bone deformity present from birth, or it may be acquired by injury over an athlete's lifetime. It is most often present in women and is related to shoe wear with rigid heels or heel counters. Individuals with a prominent protrusion of the heel bone are also susceptible to an inflammation in the heel area.

Treating Haglund's Deformity

The focus of treatment should start with reducing the painful pressure on the bump. In mild cases, a change of shoes will solve the problem and allow the irritation to heal. Changing to shoes with a lower or softer heel counter or a heel counter that is notched for the Achilles tendon can help. A heel pad can lift the heel up above the part of the heel counter that is rubbing on the bump. Icing the painful area can help, followed by warm water soaks. Anti-inflammatories can be taken to reduce the pain. If this condition becomes unbearable during an event, cutting a notch or slice into the heel counter can relieve some of the pressure off the bump.

Surgery to remove the excess bone may be necessary in extreme cases. Cortisone injections are not recommended due to the area's proximity to the Achilles tendon.

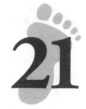

Toe Problems

"While we all have toes, some are better than others," says Herb Hedgecock, humorously relating the anatomy of his feet.

"I have ugly feet. My mother and father stuck me with an "ugly foot gene," which was a cruel thing to do. Sometimes I look at the perfect feet that others were blessed with and wonder what the hell I did to deserve Morton's toe and doublewides. The first place I get blisters is on my short fourth toe that curls under the long third monster. And the right foot does this even more. The second place is on the big toe and this seems to happen because the second toe is so damned long and the big toe curves in causing them to rub. Since the second and fourth toes are so out-of-proportion, then this seems to cause toes 1, 3, and 5 to also get in on the act. Ergo, toe blisters near the toenails; but who needs ten toenails?"

Just as varied as the many shapes and types of toes are problems associated with them. This chapter will cover the whole gamut of common toe ailments, but first, a word about basic toenail care.

The Basics: Toenail Trimming

In all the years I have been patching feet, I have observed that untrimmed toenails are the number one cause of problems leading to toe blisters and black nails. Socks will catch on nails that are too long or that have rough edges. This puts pressure on the nail bed. Nails that are too long are also prone to pressure from a toe box that is too short or too low.

TIP: The True Meaning of Buff

Elisabeth Archambault has a great toenail tip: "Consider getting a nail buffer (available for a couple of bucks in drugstore cosmetic departments) and buffing them to a shine. Smoothing out the natural ridges is one more way to reduce friction. I'm convinced this helps socks to last longer, too."

Toenails should be trimmed regularly, straight across the nail—never rounded at the corners. Leave an extra bit of nail on the outside corner of the big toe to avoid an ingrown toenail. After trimming toenails, use a nail file to smooth the top of the nail down toward the front of the toe and remove any rough edges. If you draw your finger from the skin in front of the toe up across the nail and can feel a rough edge, the nail can be filed smoother or trimmed a bit shorter. Remember though, the shorter you trim your nails, the greater the likelihood that you will experience an ingrown toenail. Conversely, nails that are too long can rub against the front of your shoes and catch on your socks, which can lead to a black toenail, wear holes in your socks, cut into other toes, and crack the nail when you run downhill. Shoes that are too tight in the forefoot or too short can cause the nail to press into the sides of the toe.

Black Toenails

The technical name for the runner's black toenail, *subungal hematoma,* describes simply a blood-filled swelling under the nail. This common occurrence is caused by the trauma of the toe or toes repetitively bumping against the front of the shoe. Individuals with Morton's toe are most susceptible to experiencing black toenails. The nail becomes discolored and usually has associated pain. Most often the nail bed turns dark, almost black or blue because of the blood. Some athletes tell of losing their nails after the nail bed has turned a whitish color.

Many runners are simply prone to black toenails. The best means of preventing black toenails is to wear shoes with a generous toe box and the proper length for your feet. Paul Vorwerk used to think shoes should fit tight "like a surgeon's glove," but after losing nails on his big toes, he now runs in shoes with good toe space. Some runners cut slits in their shoe's toe box or cut out a portion of the toe box to gain relief. Jim Winne, who has perpetually black toenails, reports that "when I have any toenails at all, I use moleskin." His strategy is to cut a piece of moleskin slightly larger than the nail area, put it on the nail, and round the edges. Use an alcohol wipe on the nail before applying and be sure the moleskin does not rub on adjoining toes. Duct tape and Elastikon tape would also work.

Treating Black Toenails

If there is no pain from the black toenail, no action may be necessary. If the pain and pressure increases, the pressure must be relieved. To relieve pressure from a black toenail, use one of the following methods, depending on the look of the toenail. The treatment may have to be repeated several times. Although the two methods below might sound painful, they are usually not. The blood has separated the nail from the nail bed and is a barrier between the nail and the live skin underneath.

- If the discoloration does not extend to the end of the toenail, swab the nail with an alcohol wipe, and use a small drill bit or hypodermic needle to gently drill a hole in the nail with light pressure and rolling the needle/bit back and forth between your thumb and fingers. The blood will ooze through the hole. Keep slight pressure on the nail bed to help expel the built-up blood. Stopping too soon will cause the blood to clot in the hole and the problem will reoccur.

- An alternative method is to use a match to heat a paper clip and gently penetrate the nail with the heated point. The heat in this method can cauterize the blood and stop the flow of blood out from under the nail. Press on the nail to expel the blood.

If the discoloration extends to the end of the toenail, use a sterile pin or needle to penetrate the skin under the nail and release the pressure. Holding slight pressure on the nail bed will help expel the blood.

Care must be taken to prevent a secondary bacterial infection through the hole in the nail or at the end of the nail by using an antibiotic ointment and covering the site with a Band-Aid. Loss of the nail usually follows in the months ahead. The new nail will begin growing, pushing up the old nail, and may come in looking odd. Dr. David Hannaford, a podiatrist, tells of patients who come to see him thinking they "have cancer because their nails are growing in funny looking." Do not be concerned about the process unless an infection develops. Remember, it can take six to nine months for a new nail to grow in completely.

You may find relief by wearing a metatarsal pad, a small circular pad that pushes up the ball of the foot and drops the toes down, which takes pressure off the toenails. Contact Hapad (**www.hapad.com**) for information on these pads.

Athletes who have frequent problems with black toenails often choose to have them surgically removed. Tim Jantz, a podiatrist, describes the process of removing a toenail:

After the toe is numbed, the nail is removed and the growth plate is treated with 89 percent phenol (some use sodium hydroxide) to destroy the growth plate. The area is then rinsed with alcohol and dressed with an antibiotic and a dressing. The usual post-operation care is daily soaks and dressing with a topical antibiotic and a Band-Aid for approximately four weeks, sometimes longer. The toe has endured a chemical burn and so heals by draining. It can have a raw feeling for a week or so, and I wouldn't want to stub it or have anyone step on it for a few weeks. You may also want to wear roomy shoes or sandals for a week. The procedure is about 95 percent successful. An option is to find a doctor that uses a laser, but the only difference is higher cost.

If you are prone to black toenails and have tried all the options to prevent them, consult a podiatrist about nail removal.

Hammertoes, Claw Toes & Mallet Toes

Hammertoes are toes that are contracted at the toe's middle joint, making the toe bend upward at its center and forcing the tip of the toe downward. The ligaments and tendons have tightened and are forcing the toe's to curl. This can lead to severe pressure and pain. Blisters or corns may form at the top bend in the toe and calluses at the ends of the toes. Hammertoes can occur in any toe, except the big toe. There are two types of hammertoes— rigid and flexible. A rigid toe has no ability to move, but in a flexible toe, the joint can be moved. Hammertoes are typically the result of a muscle imbalance that causes the ligaments and tendons to tighten. Individuals with flat feet, high arches, and Morton's toe are prone to hammertoes.

Claw toes are similar to hammertoes except they are contracted down at the middle joint and up at the joint at the ball of the foot. *Mallet toes* are contracted at the end joint only. Causes and treatments are the same as for hammer toes.

Treating Hammertoes, Claw Toes & Mallet Toes

Be sure your footwear has a high and broad toe box. This usually allows the other toes additional room so there is less friction against the individual toes. For toes that are flexible, toe crests or splints that straighten the toe can sometimes be used. Gel caps or toe shields that slide over the toes can protect the toes from friction.

Strengthening exercises can help keep toes flexible. Practice picking up marbles off a carpeted floor with your toes. Release and repeat 20 times. Put a large, sturdy rubber band around all five toes. Spread your toes outward and hold for 5 seconds, then release. Repeat 10 times.

Pamela Adams, a chiropractor, offers another alternative:

Chiropractors who specialize in sports rehab and extremity adjusting may be able to help. Even yoga for feet or a course of Rolfing (which eliminates scar tissue) may help. Tendons can shorten, tendons can lengthen. Why not try conservative approaches while saving up for surgery? You may be pleasantly surprised. I've had patients with bunions, hammertoes, and overlapping, curly and otherwise mis-aligned toes. They have had varying degrees of success using one or a combination of the three approaches I've suggested. Unless the problem is congenital, or due to an injury such as a fracture, most toe problems come from faulty alignment and biomechanics, poor shoes, and poor form during activity. I always suggest surgery as a last, not first, choice. Meanwhile, go barefoot at home and wear shoes that allow your toes to spread out when you toe off.

Adventure racer Steve Daniel's three outer toes on each foot curl up under the others—towards the big toe. When he did the Primal Quest 2003, he decided to go with what he thought was the best combination for his feet—Injinji toe socks and pretaping each toe at the joints and around any blis-ter-prone areas with Leukotape. Even with these measures, his little toe felt like it had been beaten with a hammer. That's obviously because it was pounded the whole time under the other toes. Steve talked to his podiatrist and was told surgery was his best option.

HAMMERTOES, CLAW TOES & MALLET TOES

Assorted products are available in your local drug store and pharmacy, among them Dr. Scholl's Hammertoe Pads and Gel Toe Shields or Toe Caps for cushioning the toes. Other products include the following:

FOOTSMART carries the Silicone Toe Crest that fits over one toe and "nestles" under the hammertoe for support while relieving pressure and friction. The Toe Straightener properly aligns hammertoes (also available in a double toe model). The Gel Toe Separator and Spreader may also provide relief. **FootSmart Products, (800) 870-7149, www.footsmart.com**

HAPAD offers PediFix Visco-Gel Toe Caps, Hammertoe Cushions, Toe Cushions, and Toe Spreader. **Hapad, (800) 544-2723, www.hapad.com**

Corrective surgery may be the best option, but as Steve found out, it is expensive. There are often three surgical choices: cut the tendons on the bottom of the toes; cut the tendons, fuse the joints, and put titanium pins through the toes; or cut the tendons and then add some tendons on the top side of the toe to draw the toe "up" and out. Each has its pros and cons. Your orthopedic surgeon is the best person to explain each procedure and help you make an intelligent choice.

Ingrown Toenails

Ingrown toenails, most common to the big toe, may cause infection and require medical attention. One or both sides of your toenail may grow into the flesh of the toe. The result is a reddened, irritated, and swollen toe that is sensitive to any degree of pressure. These are usually very painful and require immediate attention. Increased redness, pain, and tenderness to the touch can indicate an infection. Toes are typically in a warm and moist environment, and bacteria can quickly take hold. The most common cause of an ingrown toenail is improper nail trimming (see "The Basics: Toenail Trimming" above).

Sometimes trauma from a stubbed toe or someone stepping on your toe can cause the nail to be jammed into the skin. Repeated trauma, such as the pounding to which athletes typically subject their feet, also can lead to ingrown toenails. The medical term for an ingrown toenail is *onychocryptosis*.

Treating Ingrown Toenails

Soak your foot in warm water or Epsom salts two to three times a day to reduce the infection. Do not poke at the ingrown nail. If you cannot trim the nail yourself, check with your orthopedist or podiatrist. An ignored ingrown toenail can become seriously infected. Apply a layer of antibiotic cream to help reduce inflammation and cover with a Band-Aid.

Rich Schick, a physician's assistant, recommends the following method to care for an ingrown nail:

> File the entire top surface of the nail from near the cuticle to the tip until you get it as thin as possible. A regular nail file will work, but a medium-grade metal file is much quicker. This weakens the nail.

Then soak the foot in hot water for about thirty minutes to soften the nail, further weakening the nail. Then use a cuticle trimmer (available in most drugstore beauty departments) to free the ingrown portion. Do not attempt to work from the tip towards the base. Come from the side, and a little towards the base of the toe and use the "wings" of the instrument to lift and free the ingrown segment. As you continue forward, the trimmer will often cut the piece off. If not, snip it with a nail clipper. I prefer a small pair of wire cutters for the task.

Assorted products are available in your local drugstore and pharmacy. In addition to ingrown toenail files and toenail softening cream, here are few specialty products:

- The Barrel Nipper, a long-handled nail clippers made for thick, tough, curved nails
- Dr. Scholl's Ingrown Toenail Relief Strips
- Toe Caps and Jelly Tips from Hapad (**www.hapad.com**) or Bunheads (**www.bunhead.com**) to cover and protect the nail

Morton's Toe

Morton's toe is a common problem in which the second toe (next to the big toe) is longer than the big toe. The first metatarsal (of the big toe) is shorter than normal, and this makes the second toe appear longer than it actually is. This is usually a hereditary condition. The repeated pressure of the longer second toe against the front of the shoe or boot may traumatize the nail. If a hematoma develops under the nail, the nail will change color and may fall off. Because of the excessive pressure on the second metatarsal head in the forefoot, Morton's toe is often associated with metatarsalgia.

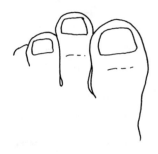

Those with Morton's toe have a second toe that extends beyond the big toe.

Treating Morton's Toe

To get a good fit, look for shoes or boots with a high and wide toe box. It may be necessary to use a shoe or boot a half size to a size larger than normal in order to have space for the longer first toe. The use of a nonslippery insole will keep the foot from sliding forward. Look for an insole with a good heel cup, an arch that fits your foot, and a surface material that grips the foot and sock. Some runners will cut a slit over or on either side of the toe to relieve pressure. Another option is to cut out a small piece of the toe box over the toe. Orthotics may also provide relief. Surgery is usually a last resort.

If you find a blister or corn starting at the top of the toe, use a Gel Cap or tape to protect the area. If you begin to experience pain at the base of the toe, a pad might help. Use a U-shaped pad and position the cut out area at the site of the pain. To find the right position, first make a mark at the sore area with marking pen. Then slide your foot inside your shoe and step down to transfer the ink onto the insole. Stick the pad to the insole with the opening towards the toes.

FOOTSMART carries Silicone Gel Caps and Digi-Cushions to cushion the toe, and Felt and Silicone Callus Cushions for the base of the toe pain. **FootSmart Products, (800) 870-7149, www.footsmart.com**

Overlapping Toes

Sometimes toes will overlap other toes. This can occur with any of your toes and cause extreme irritation. Overlapping toes typically involve one toe lying on top of an adjacent toe. The fifth toe is the most affected digit with overlapping toes. Underlapping toes usually involve the fourth and fifth toes. The cause of overlapping and underlapping toes is unknown. Many experts suspect they are caused by an imbalance in the small muscles of the foot.

Treating Overlapping Toes

Custom-made orthotics may help align the toes. Off-the-shelf orthotics commonly found in drugstores and sports stores will generally not help this condition. A podiatrist can make the correct type of orthotic. Shoes with a high and wide toe box can give toes the space they need. Gel toe straighteners, toe caps, and toe combs can be used on and between toes. Pamela Adams, a chiropractor, in the section above on hammertoes, offers an option worth considering. Chiropractic toe adjustments may be help as well. If the condition is painful and causes problems when participating in sports, consult with your podiatrist to determine your options.

FOOTSMART carries the Gel Toe Separators and Spreader. **FootSmart Products, (800) 870-7149, www.footsmart.com**

Stubbed Toes

Occasionally we stub our toes badly, and this can result in a hematoma, a bruise, or even a fracture. Stubbed toes are more common in running shoes than in hiking boots. Stubbing a toe on a rock or tree root can be very painful. Check the toe for discoloration that can indicate a deep bruise or a fracture. There may be a laceration into the nail bed or into the toe itself.

Treating Stubbed Toes

Treatment includes buddy taping, icing the toe (a cold stream will also work), and elevating the foot, and wearing a firm-soled shoe or boot. Buddy taping provides support and a limited degree of immobilization to the toe. It involves lightly taping the injured toe to the toe next to it after placing a piece of cotton between toes (never tape skin to skin). See the chapter "Cold & Heat Therapy" for information on making the most of icing techniques. A firm-soled shoe will keep the toe from bending, providing additional immobilization. For elevation to be effective, the injured toe should be above the level of the heart and iced.

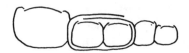

Buddy taping as seen from the front.

If it heals in a few days, it is probably not fractured. On the other hand, if the injury does not respond to treatment, medical treatment and an X-ray may be necessary (see the section on fractures, page 239). A doctor may have you wear an orthopedic shoe, a wooden-soled shoe that does not allow the foot to bend. If the toe is fractured, expect a healing time of four to six weeks.

If you stub your toe and the nail is bent backwards, it's important to prevent the toenail from catching on your sock and tearing off. Wrap either a Band-Aid or tape around the toe to hold the toenail in place. The use of an antibiotic ointment under the nail will help prevent infection. Trimming off any loose parts of the nail will help prevent the nail from lifting off further.

Toenail Fungus

Toenails infected with a fungus usually become thick and deformed. The infection may cause the nail to have a brown, white or yellowish discoloration. The nail may become brittle and give the appearance of debris under the nail.

Treating Toenail Fungus

Usually doctors will prescribe a strong medication to destroy the fungus. Medication may include oral antifungal pills or a medicated nail polish. If you are prescribed an oral medication, be sure to discuss its side effects with your doctor. In extreme cases, nail removal is necessary.

Tree tea oil is often used for nail fungus. For best results, apply a few drops to the affected nail and skin around the nail two to three times daily. Dab it on with a cotton swab or ball. Hold it in place with a bandage or tape. As well as killing the fungi, it helps relieve the associated itching. Test a drop or two on your skin to be sure you are not allergic to the oil. The oil can be found in your local drugstore or pharmacy.

Another nail treatment that has been used with success is Vicks Vapo-Rub. Trim the nail back as far as possible and scrape out as much of the loose nail as possible. Apply a thin coat of VapoRub over the nail and in the space underneath. Cover the nail with a Band-Aid. Repeat daily every morning and evening, and over a few months the fungus will die out and a new nail will grow in.

Once you have had a nail fungus, you are more susceptible to its return. Since the fungus can be spread between to other people, wear shower clogs in public locker rooms and showers.

Turf Toe

Turf toe is pain at the base of the big toe where it connects to the ball of the foot. It is usually caused from either jamming the toe, or pushing off repeatedly when running or jumping. There may also be an associated stiffness and swelling. This injury is especially common among athletes who play on the hard surface of artificial turf. Football and soccer players are most susceptible to it because of all their running and jumping.

The injury is actually a tear of the capsule that surrounds the joint at the base of the toe. Tearing this joint capsule can be extremely painful. The tearing of the joint capsule can lead to instability and even dislocation of the joint at the base of the toe.

Robin Fry, a physician's assistant, remembers during an ultramarathon in 1993, he was "running away from the fire-tower aid station. Suddenly, a terrible pain shot out from my left foot and a swear word or two shot out from my mouth. I had slammed my left great toe into an unseen remnant of a small shrub or tree, barely protruding from the rough trail surface." Years later in 2001, her podiatrist performed surgery to repair the toe, which by then was very deviated laterally, and was crowding the second toe and pushing it into the third toe. After a period of recovery, Robin reports, "I do get some occasional aching in the repaired toe, but it generally stays at a tolerable level and only hurts after some very long, hard efforts. The long-crowded toes of my left foot are gradually resuming a normal alignment. I rarely take any NSAIDS. I have been taking daily CosaminDS, a glucosamine and chondroitin-sulfate supplement, since early January. And I am back to my old training ways."

Treating Turf Toe

The common treatment consists of resting the sore toe, icing the area, and elevating the foot. An anti-inflammatory medication may be prescribed by your doctor. Avoid playing your sport for about three weeks to allow the joint capsule to heal. When returning to play, you may have to wear a special toe support to protect the joint capsule. Like many injuries, the condition can recur and the rate of rehabilitation can slow with each occurrence. As Robin found out, surgery may be necessary in extreme cases or when the initial injury heals incorrectly.

HAPAD DANCER PADS fit under the ball of the foot with a cutout encompassing the big toe joint to relieve the pain under the first metatarsal joint. The coiled, springlike wool fibers provide firm and resilient support as they mold and shape to the foot. **Hapad, (800) 544-2723, www.hapad.com**

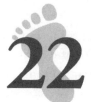

Forefoot Problems

Four conditions commonly affect the front of the foot (the forefoot): bunions, metatarsalgia, Morton's neuroma, and sesamoiditis. Any of them can be bothersome and painful, but when they happen to an athlete, they can make enjoying your sport more challenging.

Bunions

Bunions are one of the most common deformities of the forefoot. A bunion is a bump caused by enlarged bone and tissue at the outer base of the big toe where the joint angles inward toward the other toes. A displacement of the first metatarsal bone toward the midline (center) of the body and a simultaneous displacement of the big toe away from the midline (and towards the smaller toes) cause this bump to appear. Over time, the big toe can come to rest under, or occasionally over, the second toe. The bony bump is a form of arthritis. The medical term for bunions is *hallux valgus.*

The deformity gives you a wide foot and causes a weakening and sagging of the arch. The motion of the joint and shoe pressure can cause pain. There may be corns on the adjacent sides of the first and second toes. A callus may develop over the bunion, and bursitis can form between the skin and the bunion bone.

A similar bump at the outer base of the fifth (small) toe is called a *bunionette*. These are formed when the little toe moves inward toward the big toe. Bunionettes are sometimes called Taylor's bunions.

Bunions are caused by various factors. An abnormal pronated foot that rolls inward is one of the most common causes. Other causes include a family history of bunions, wearing shoes that are too narrow-toed, and limb length discrepancy. Individuals with flat feet are more prone to bunions, calluses, and hammertoes.

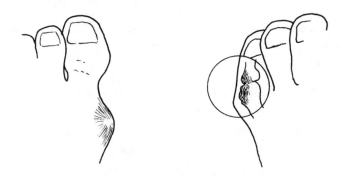

Bunion (left) and bunionette (right).

Treating Bunions

Be sure your shoes are wide and deep enough in the forefoot and toe box. If you overpronate, try an arch support or orthotic to reduce the overpronation. Bunion discomfort may be relieved with wider shoes, pads between the big and first toes, arch supports, and warm soaks. Wearing shoes or boots that are tapered in the toe area can cause bunions to worsen. Check the foot-care section of your local drugstore for a current selection of bunion relief products. If there is an inflammation of the bunion, take an anti-inflammatory medication, elevate the foot, and apply ice three times a day, 15 minutes at a time. For information on cold and heat therapy techniques, see page 306. Surgery may be necessary in extreme cases.

A full-service shoe shop or a pedorthist should be able to modify a boot to soften a pressure point or stretch a portion of the leather. This may relieve pressure on bunions, corns, and calluses.

To relieve pressure on the painful area, try one of these lacing techniques. Use one pair of laces (that is, two laces) per shoe. Lace one through the bottom half of the eyelets, and tie it loosely. Lace the other through the top half of the eyelets, and tie it more tightly than the bottom lace. A second technique is to lace the first few loops loosely, tie a knot, and then lace the rest of the way up the shoe. Both methods allow a looser fit in the forefoot.

BUNION PRODUCTS

Assorted bunion products are available in your local drugstore and pharmacy, among them Dr. Scholl's Bunion Cushion Pads and Hapad's Daytime Bunion Cushion.

ENGO PERFORMANCE PATCHES are made of a thin fabric-film composite that can greatly reduce friction in targeted locations within your footwear. The patches add a slick, slippery surface to the inside of your shoe where the bunion rubs. Patches come in three sizes: small ovals, large ovals, and sheets, and they can be trimmed for a custom fit. Each patch is extremely durable, lasting anywhere from several weeks to several months. **Tamarack Habilitation Technologies Inc., (763) 795-0057, www.goengo.com**

FOOTSMART carries the Gel Toe Separators and Spreader, Bunion Comforter, and Hydrogel Bunion Guard. **FootSmart Products, (800) 870-7149, www.footsmart.com**

Metatarsalgia

Metatarsalgia is pain underneath the metatarsal heads of the foot. It typically occurs when one of the metatarsal heads collapses and points downward. Typically the second metatarsal head is affected, but it can also be at the third or fourth metatarsal heads. You may feel like there is a small stone in your shoe, or you may feel pain, a burning sensation, or swelling at the ball of the foot. By pressing up slightly on each metatarsal head, you can usually identify the painful area. Typically the metatarsal head that is lower then the others is causing the pain and pressure. There will often be a callus at the pressure point. As we age, the fat pads on the bottoms of our feet tend to thin out and our feet become more susceptible to this problem. Metatarsalgia is often associated with Morton's Foot.

Shoes that are too narrow in the forefoot or laced too tight over the forefoot area can cause all of these problems. To see how the pressure in a narrow shoe affects the metatarsals, try this simple test. Grasp your foot around the base of the toes and squeeze gently. See how it forces the metatarsals downward (on the bottom of the foot) and results in increased impact to the area with each step. For proper prevention, start with shoes that fit correctly and use good lacing techniques (for more on these topics, see the chapters "The Magic of Fit," page 31, and "Lacing Options," page 136).

METATARSALGIA PRODUCTS

FOOTSMART carries a Silicone Ball-of-Foot Cushion and Metatarsal Pad that redistributes pressure on the metatarsal heads. **FootSmart Products, (800) 870-7149, www.footsmart.com**

HAPAD makes several pads to relieve metatarsal pain. Metatarsal pads relieve the pain of metatarsalgia and Morton's neuroma. Metatarsal bars relieve pressure on the ball of the foot that causes painful calluses and forefoot irritations. Metatarsal Cookies provide simple metatarsal arch cushioning. The coiled, springlike wool fibers provide firm and resilient support as they mold and shape to the foot. **Hapad, (800) 544-2723, www.hapad.com**

SPENCO'S METATARSAL ARCH CUSHION is made for the ball of the foot. **Spenco Medical Corporation, (800) 877-3626, www.spenco.com**

VISCOPED INSOLES are made from a noncompressible viscoelastic material with areas of softer density in the raised metatarsal head pad and heel areas. The Viscoped S insole is made with bar of softer silicon in the metatarsal and heel areas. The insoles reduce shock throughout the entire length of the insole, distribute pressure evenly, and are made to relieve pain associated with metatarsalgia and Morton's neuroma. **Bauerfeind USA, (800) 423-3405, www.bauerfeindusa.com**

Treating Metatarsalgia

A cushioned metatarsal pad can provide relief from metatarsalgia. If a pad does not help, try cutting a small hole in the insole under the painful metatarsal head. Some metatarsal pads are made in a sleeve that wraps around the foot, and this design may cause problems during sports. To find the right position for a pad, first make a mark at the sore area with marking pen. Then slide your foot inside your shoe and step down to transfer the ink onto the insole. Stick the pad to the insole with the opening towards the toes.

Wearing shoes with a wide forefoot and high and wide toe box is also recommended. An orthotic may be necessary.

Morton's Neuroma

Morton's neuroma is pain associated with a nerve inflammation usually affecting the third and fourth toes. It will sometimes be felt between the second and third toes. The nerves running between the metatarsal heads and the toes have become inflamed and irritated as they are squeezed at the base of the toes. The painful, swollen nerve is called a neuroma. There is typically tingling, burning, or a pins-and-needles sensation that radiates to the end of the toes. Some people describe the sensation as walking on a pebble. If you press with your thumb at the base of your fourth toe and feel pain, you could have a neuroma. If untreated, scar tissue forms around the nerve and it becomes more painful.

This condition can be caused by a shoe's tight toe box that compresses the forefoot or by the nerves being pressured by the metatarsal heads and the bases of the toes. Sports that place a significant amount of pressure on the forefoot area can cause inflammation of the nerves. As we walk or run, we come up onto our toes, and this motion can cause the ligaments supporting the metatarsal bones to compress the nerve

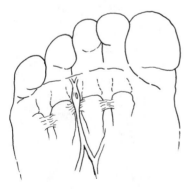

Inflammation of a nerve, indicating Morton's neuroma.

between the toes. Limiting your activities for a few days may be enough to allow the inflammation to subside.

Treating Morton's Neuroma

Treatments include applying ice to the pain area, an injection of anti-inflammatory medication, wider shoes, a more cushioned insole, and metatarsal pads that take pressure off the metatarsal heads. The pad reduces forefoot pressure and spreads the toes, which can relieve the pain. To find the right position for a pad, first make a mark at the sore area with a marking pen. Then slide your foot inside your shoe and step down to transfer the ink onto the insole. Stick the pad to the insole with the opening towards the toes. Massaging the foot usually helps to relieve the pain. Using icing techniques from the "Cold & Heat Therapy" chapter can help reduce pain and inflammation.

If you overpronate, the metatarsal bones have more movement, which can irritate the nerves running between the metatarsal heads. In this case, wearing firm motion-control shoes may help. Relief may also be gained by inserting a piece of lamb's wool between the toes. The use of an orthotic may be indicated. Bursitis, bunions, or arthritis may also cause metatarsal pain.

TIP: Strengthening Exercises

Toe exercises help to strengthen and tighten the metatarsal arch and stretch the tendons on top of the toes. Practice picking up marbles off a carpeted floor with your toes. Or put a towel on the floor and use your toes to scrunch up the towel and pick it up.

Your podiatrist or orthopedist can help identify the cause of the pain and make recommendations on how to treat the problems. A course of oral anti-inflammatory medication may be suggested. Cortisone injections are sometimes used to control the pain. Serious neuromas may require surgery to release or remove the affected nerve.

To relieve pressure on the metatarsal heads and forefoot, try different lacing techniques (see the methods described in the "Bunions" section above). With these methods the metatarsal heads are not squeezed by the pressure of normal lacing. The "Lacing" chapter describes other lacing techniques.

MORTON'S NEUROMA PRODUCTS

FOOTSMART offers a Silicone Forefoot Insole, a Forefoot Pad with Metatarsal Dome, and a Plantar Cushion. **FootSmart Products, (800) 870-7149, www.footsmart.com**

HAPAD makes several pads for neuromas (see "Metatarsalgia Products" above).

SPENCO'S METATARSAL ARCH CUSHION is made for the ball of the foot. **Spenco Medical Corporation, (800) 877-3626, www.spenco.com**

VISCOPED INSOLES may prove helpful (see "Metatarsalgia Products" page 287).

Sesamoiditis

Sesamoiditis is an inflammation of the two little bones beneath the ball of the foot under the joint that moves the big toe. These two sesamoid bones can become bruised and inflamed, resulting in either sharp, constant pain or pain that occurs with movement of the big toe. The bones can also fracture, resulting in sudden, intense pain and the inability to bear weight on the foot.

Athletes involved in sports that place repetitive and excessive pressure on the forefoot area can experience sesamoid pain. Shoes with poor cushioning that offer inadequate protection against rocks can cause trauma to the sesamoid bones.

Rich Schick, a physician's assistant, points out that the sesamoid under the first metatarsal is often composed of several small bones.

If the bones on an X-ray were smooth appearing with no rough or jagged edges, this is likely the situation. Even if it is a fracture, these bones only act as shock absorbers in the first place. One can continue to run with nothing to fear but pain. I high-centered on a sharp rock some years back and fractured mine. On X-ray there were two pieces like half moons with the round side smooth and the straight sides jagged as one would expect if you broke a round object in half. The literature said that these fractures could lead to chronic pain and the fragments could need to be surgically removed. As this "worse case" didn't seem all that frightening, I opted to train and race as normal. The thing bothered me for about a year, but for the last several years has given me no pain at all.

These two little bones can became a major problem. The ball of Lyal Holmberg's left foot became painful during a short 5-mile run. An X-ray showed the sesamoid bone was broken into three pieces. Lyal reports that "as I continued running, the foot was killing me and caused a tilt towards the right, putting a strain on my left hip." A walking-type boot and an anti-inflammatory was prescribed for two weeks, followed by the use of a small "dancer's" pad behind the ball of his foot. Lyal says, "If I can walk and run without pain, then the problem is solved. If not, I may need surgery to correct the problem."

Treating Sesamoiditis

The use of soft pads or insoles can help. You can also cut a small hole in your insole under the sesamoid bones. Loosely lacing the forefoot of your shoes, as described in the "Bunion" section above, can help relieve pressure on the sesamoid area. Using icing techniques from the "Cold & Heat Therapy" chapter can help reduce pain and inflammation.

Buddy taping the big toe to the second toe or toes next to it for stabilization will limit movement of the toe. A small piece of gauze, cotton, or tissue between the taped toes will prevent skin breakdown if the tape is on for any great length of time. A firm-soled shoe will help keep the toe in line and the foot-toe joint stable.

SESAMOIDITIS PRODUCTS

HAPAD DANCER PADS fit under the ball of the foot with a cutout encompassing the big toe joint to relieve calluses and the painful irritations of sesamoiditis. The coiled, springlike wool fibers provide firm and resilient support as they mold and shape to the foot. **Hapad, (800) 544-2723, www.hapad.com**

VISCOPED INSOLES may provide relief (see "Metatarsalgia Products" above).

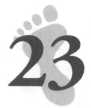

Numb Toes & Feet

Numb feet are usually caused by either transient parasthesia or peripheral neuropathy. Though both are bothersome, the first is usually temporary while the second can be very debilitating. Another form of numbness that is fairly common is Raynaud's syndrome.

Transient Parasthesia

Transient parasthesia is a temporary nerve-compression that can be caused by a gradual buildup of fluids in your feet during extended on-your-feet activity. As the feet swell and blood flow decreases, nerves become compressed. During the compression, the nerves do not receive the oxygen-rich blood they need, resulting in numbness and/or tingling. Tight shoes and/or tightly laced shoes contribute to the problem. Shoes with poor cushioning, coupled with a heavy, pounding gait, can also be a factor.

Ultrarunner and adventure racer Ginny La Forma has battled this numbness in her toes on many occasions. After the Hardrock 100-Mile Run, it lasted a few weeks, but after the EcoChallenge it lasted over a year. She also suffers from Morton's neuromas

If the problem continues after your activity has stopped, consider changing to more cushioned shoes and changing insoles and arch supports. There may be some lymph system breakdown in the foot caused by microtrauma. If the problem persists, consult a sports specialist.

Information Resources for Transient Parasthesia

THE NEUROPATHY ASSOCIATION, www.neuropathy.org

THE NEUROPATHY TRUST, www.neuropathy-trust.org

NUMB TOES AND ACHING SOLES is a must read for anyone experiencing peripheral neuropathy. Written by John A. Senneff, who suffers from peripheral neuropathy, the book deals with this disorder from the patient's perspective. **Medpress, July 1999, ISBN 0967110718**

Peripheral Neuropathy

Peripheral neuropathy is a painful nerve condition that can manifest itself as a burning sensation in the feet but which sometimes will appear as a cold sensation. It may start as a mild tingling in the toes and progress to searing pain. It can spread upward in the body, even to the thighs. Other symptoms might include tingling, prickling, or numbness; the sensation of having an "invisible sock" on your feet; a sharp jabbing or electric-type pain; extreme sensitivity to touch; muscle weakness; and a loss of balance or coordination.

The pain results from damage to peripheral nerves that can come from a myriad of causes. A partial list of causes includes diabetes, kidney or liver disease, an underactive thyroid, viral and bacterial infections, vitamin deficiencies, and pressure on a single nerve, although often, no cause is identified.

Ken Reed, an ultrarunner who discovered a year and one half ago that he had peripheral neuropathy, shares this story. His condition started with a tingling in three of his left foot toes in the summer of 1998 that later turned to numbness. When the numbness progressed to shooting pains and aches that fall, he sought medical advice. By the spring of 1999 it had progressed to pains in his lower legs, with the numbness also moving upwards. Ken reports that when his feet are cold, they constantly ache, buzz, and feel numb. He has resolved to managing the pain and discomfort, and hope for a miracle cure.

Treating Peripheral Neuropathy

Treatment often depends on the cause and symptoms of the neuropathy. It can be frustrating to treat, particularly if no reversible cause is identified. Typical treatments include over-the-counter or prescribed pain relievers for mild symptoms, tricyclic antidepressants for burning pain, antiseizure medications for jabbing pain, or other drugs.

Self-care treatments include proper care of your feet with loose socks and padded shoes, a semicircular hoop in bed to keep the cover off your feet, cold water soaks and skin moisturizers, massage to improve circulation and stimulate nerves, staying active, and reducing stress levels.

Raynaud's Syndrome

Raynaud's syndrome affects 5 to 10 percent of the population. The discomfort is caused by a decreased blood supply to the fingers and toes. Attacks are precipitated by exposure to cold and stress.

Although the severity, duration, and frequency of attacks vary both between individuals and over time, the primary symptoms of Raynaud's syndrome are changes in skin color. The affected areas turn white from the lack of circulation, then blue and cold, and finally numb. When the attack subsides, the affected parts may turn red and may throb, tingle, or swell.

Treating Raynaud's Syndrome

Keeping your whole body warm is a good prevention strategy. Wear wind- and water-resistant gloves and socks. Wool or wool-blend socks that retain warmth are good. Shoes that block wind and moisture are also recommended. Be sure to allow space in your footwear for thicker socks. Constriction caused by tight socks and footwear can be harmful. Keep fingers and toes dry with talcum powder. If you feel an attack coming on, get inside and warm your hands and feet.

Be careful not to injure the skin in affected areas, and treat injuries without delay. Even minor cuts and scrapes take longer to heal and may be more susceptible to infection when circulation is impaired.

If you suspect you have Raynaud's syndrome, see your physician. Doctors sometimes recommend medications to help combat this condition. The Raynaud's Association (**www.raynauds.org**) can offer help and support for this painful and frustrating condition.

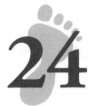

Skin Disorders

Five skin disorders commonly affect the feet: athlete's foot, calluses, corns, fissures, and plantar warts. Dealing with these conditions when they first develop will help prevent more serious problems later.

Athlete's Foot

Athlete's foot, technically called *tinea pedis,* is a skin disease caused by a fungus. The hot weather and foot perspiration that athletes typically encounter can make athlete's foot a common problem. The combination of a warm and humid environment in the shoes or boots, excessive foot perspiration, and changes in the condition of the skin combine to create a setting for the fungi of athlete's foot to begin growing. Athlete's foot usually occurs between the toes or under the arch of the foot. Typical signs and symptoms of athlete's foot include itching, dry and cracking skin, inflammation with a burning sensation, and pain. Blisters and swelling may develop if left untreated. When these blisters break, small, red areas of raw tissue are exposed. As the infection spreads, the burning and itching will increase.

Another type of tinea infection is often called "moccasin foot." In this type, a red rash spreads across the lower portion of the foot in the pattern of a moccasin. The skin in this region gradually becomes dense, white, and scaly. The use of a prescription strength antifungal cream may be required to treat this infection.

Fungus under and around the nails should be treated promptly with antifungal medications. See the "Toenail Fungus" section (page 281) for information on treating fungal infections.

Preventive measures include washing your feet daily with soap and water; drying them thoroughly, especially between the toes; wearing moisture-wicking socks; regularly changing your shoes and socks to control moisture; and the use of a good, moisture absorbing, foot powder. If you use a communal shower or bathroom after an event, or use a gym to train, avoid walking barefoot in these areas. Use thongs, shower booties, or even your shoes or boots.

Treating Athlete's Foot

Treatment includes keeping the feet clean and dry, frequent socks changes, antifungal medications, and foot powders (see the "Powders" section, page 281, for more information on choosing a foot powder). An antiperspirant may also help those with excessive foot moisture (see the "Antiperspirants for the Feet" section, page 98, for more information about these products).

Check your local drugstore or pharmacy for a complete line of athlete's foot antifungal ointments, creams, liquids, powders, and sprays. See your doctor if your feet do not respond to treatment with over-the-counter medications. If the fungus returns, alternate medications since it can sometimes build up a resistance to a particular fungicide.

To treat athlete's foot or a case of foot fungi, give tree tea oil a try. For best results, apply a few drops to the affected areas two to three times daily. Dab it on with a cotton swab or cotton ball. Hold it in place with a bandage or tape. As well as killing the fungi, it helps relive the associated itching. Test a drop or two on your skin to be sure you are not allergic to the oil. The oil can be found in your local drugstore or pharmacy.

Other over-the-counter antifungal creams or solutions commonly available in your local drugstore and pharmacy include Dr. Scholl's Fungal Nail Revitalizer and Fungi Solution, Clotrimazole, Lamisi. Lotrimin, Micatin, Tinactin, and Tolnaftate are all common. Zeasorb-AF is available as a powder and a lotion/powder combination.

Calluses

A *callus* is an abnormal amount of dead, thickened skin caused by recurring pressure and friction, called hyperkeratosis, usually on the sole of the foot, most often on the heels, the balls of the feet, or the bottom of the toes. They may be yellowish in color, layered, or even scaly due to excessive dryness. Calluses can form over any bony prominence. Calluses are never normal— they are signs of poor biomechanics or ill-fitting footgear. If it is a footgear problem, this needs to be identified and remedied. Unfortunately most biomechanical problems are things we need to learn to live with. Calluses become a problem when they become thick enough to interfere with the normal elasticity of the skin or to act like a foreign body on the foot.

A common callus is called intractable plantar keratosis; this is a localized callus buildup at or near the metatarsal heads on the ball of the foot. Calluses are caused by a number of factors: poorly aligned metatarsal bones in the fore-foot, an abnormal gait, flat or high-arched feet, excessively long metatarsal bones, and a loss of the fat pads on the underside of the foot. Individuals with flat feet are more prone to calluses, bunions, and hammertoes.

Unless the callus is troublesome, most people tend to forget about them. Your body has made the callus as protection from pressure at those points with little natural fat or padding. To keep painful calluses from returning, you must correct the biomechanical problem that prompted their growth in the first place. Some calluses may have a deep-seated core, called *nucleation,* that can be painful to pressure.

Calluses will continue to grow as they toughen. This can interfere with the fit of your shoes—which in turn can cause a blister—one way or another. The time to treat calluses is before an event. Should you develop blisters under-neath the tough, hardened surface of a callus, it will usually form deep in the foot, which makes it hard to treat. Once you have experienced a deep blister, you are likely to work hard to rid your feet of their thick calluses. Some degree of toughened skin is fine, but be careful of too-callused skin. The section "Deep Blisters" (see page 225) discusses treating these problem blisters.

Treating Calluses

Gently grasp some normal skin on your foot and roll it between your thumb and forefinger. Notice how supple it is. Now attempt to roll the callused area in the same manner. If it is too stiff or causes discomfort, the callus is too thick and is likely to cause pain or blisters. You need to thin it down.

Soak your feet weekly in warm water with a bag of tissue-softening chamomile tea to help soften calluses. After soaking, buff with a pumice stone or callus file to remove any dead skin. After the callused skin is dry, apply your choice of cream, lotion, medication, or pads. If your skin is particularly callused, at night after applying the cream, wrap your feet with Saran Wrap to hold in the moisturizer. Socks can be worn to bed instead, but they absorb some of the moisturizer off the skin. Over several weeks, simply keep working at it until all areas are as supple as normal skin.

Ultrarunner Geraldine Wales has a tendency to get tough calluses on her feet that turn into hot spots and eventually blisters. In the evening she uses a file on the calluses and then applies moisturizing cream to keep her feet soft. Never file too deeply into a corn or callus and do not cut into them with sharp objects. A pumice stone will work as well as a file.

A cushioned insole with a good arch support can help equalize the weight load of the foot, while pads around or near the callus can relieve pressure. To relieve heel discomfort from calluses, try a heel cup or heel pad that will distribute body weight evenly across the heel. Orthotics can help relieve pressure in the callused areas of your feet. While there are a variety of callus pads sold, these are only temporary fixes. The regular use of skin moisturizers will help keep the skin soft and eliminate the thick calluses. To relieve pressure on the painful area, try different lacing techniques (see the lacing discussion in the "Bunions" section, page 284). While there are over-the-counter plantar wart removal compounds available that can also be used on corns and calluses, care must be taken in their use. These products contain salicylic acid. Follow the product's directions to avoid damaging good tissue. Do not use these products if you are a diabetic.

Assorted callus products can be found at your local drugstore and pharmacy. These include Carmol 20 and Carmol 40 Crea; Dr. Scholl's Pedicure File, Dual-Action Swedish File, Callus Reducer, Callus Cushions, and Cushlin Gel Pads; and Pretty Feet & Hands Rough Skin Remover.

CALLUS PRODUCTS

AVON'S DOUBLE ACTION FOOT FILE is 7 inches long and has a coarse side and a fine side to remove dry skin buildup and calluses. It can be used on either wet or dry skin. After filing, apply a moisturizing cream. **Avon Products, (800) FOR-AVON, www.avon.com**

BUNGA Oval Pads and Gel Pads are made from a medical-grade polymer material. **Absolute Athletics, (888) 286-4272, www.bungapads.com**

ENGO PERFORMANCE PATCHES are made of a thin fabric-film composite that can greatly reduce friction in targeted locations within your footwear. The patches can give a slick, slippery surface to the inside of your footwear or insole where calluses rub. Patches come in three sizes: small ovals, large ovals and sheets and they can be trimmed for a custom fit. Each patch is extremely durable, lasting anywhere from several weeks to several months. **Tamarack Habilitation Technologies Inc., (763) 795.0057, www.tamaracktech.com**

FOOTSMART carries a complete line of skin care products made for calluses. These products will help your feet feel softer and smoother while eliminating calluses. Total Foot Recovery Cream comes in three formulas: Original, Tree Tea Oil, and Shea Butter Formula. Callus Treatment Cream with Urethin breaks down painful, hardened skin. The Credo Callus Rasp reduces thick calluses. Callex Callus Ointment and polymer cushions and pads may also prove helpful. **FootSmart Products, (800) 870-7149, www.footsmart.com**

HAPAD offers several options for callus control. Metatarsal pads and metatarsal bars, Metatarsal Cookies, Dancer Pads with a cutout encompassing the big toe joint, heel cushions and Horseshoe Heel Cushions all reduce pressure on areas of calluses. The IPK Pad is made for intractable plantar keratosis. The coiled, springlike wool fibers provide firm and resilient support as they mold and shape to the foot. **Hapad, (800) 544-2723, www.hapad.com**

ZIM'S CRACK CREAM helps to moisturize, soothe, and soften dry, cracked, painful skin. You can choose between two formulas: a nighttime liquid or daytime cream. The creams are formulated with their unique herbal base of arnica and myrcia oil. Look for Zim's in your drugstore or pharmacy. **Perfecta Products, (800) 319-2225, www.crackcream.com**

Corns

A corn is a hard, thickened area of skin, generally on the top of, the tip of, or between the toes, usually caused by friction and pressure. A corn is usually, like a kernel of corn, round and yellowish in color. Corns on the outer surface of the toes are usually hard, while those between the toes are usually soft. The larger the corn and the more it rubs against your shoe, the more painful it becomes. Typically the corn is an inverted cone shape with

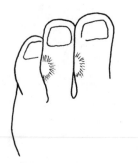

a point that can press on a nerve below, causing pain.

Corns can be caused by tight fitting socks and footwear, deformed toes, or the foot sliding around the shoe. Soft corns, caused by prominent, irregularly shaped bones and bumps, occur between the toes—soft from the perspiration in the forefoot area.

Treating Corns

Weekly warm water and Epsom salt soaks will help soften corns. Following the soak, apply a moisturizing cream and cover them with plastic wrap for 15 minutes. After removing the warp, gently buff off any dead tissue with a pumice stone.

To relieve the discomfort of corns, start with properly fitting shoes with extra room in the toe box. You can also pad around the corn with corn pads, small pieces of one of the tapes previously mentioned, or Spenco 2nd Skin. There are many types of corn pads and toe sleeves. Lamb's wool can be wrapped around the toe for cushioning.

Check the foot-care section of your local drugstore for a current selection of corn relief products. These may include pads and creams to remove the corns. If your corns persist, consult your podiatrist.

To control corns, the pressure and friction must be eliminated, usually from improper fitting shoes. To relieve pressure on the painful area, try the lacing techniques described in the Bunions section (page 284). Both methods allow a looser fit in the forefoot.

PRODUCTS FOR CORNS

Assorted corn relief products can be found at your local drugstore and pharmacy. These include Band-Aid Corn Remover, and Dr. Scholl's Corn Cushions, Moisturizing and Corn Remover Kit, and One-Step Corn Remover Pads.

BUNGA Oval Pads and Gel Pads are made from a medical-grade polymer material. **Absolute Athletics, (888) 286-4272, www.bungapads.com**

HAPAD has Metatarsal Cookies that provide simple metatarsal arch cushioning. These can relieve the pressure that causes corns and calluses and PediFix Visco-Gel Corn protectors. **Hapad, (800) 544-2723, www.hapad.com**

Fissures

Fissures often develop in the thickened callused skin on our heels, but they also occur on callused skin on the balls of the feet. These fissures can become infected, may bleed, and can split open into the deeper underlying tissues. Like many foot conditions, fissures if left untreated, can lead to infection.

Wearing sandals and going barefoot can contribute to fissures. On vacation one summer, I wore Teva's everyday. My feet were in and out of water all day. After several days of in the hot, drying sun, I had several deep fissures on one heel. I discovered how painful these cracks can become.

Treating Fissures

Using a moisturizing cream on your feet will help prevent fissures. If wearing sandals or going barefoot, use the cream morning and evening. The "Calluses" section above has information and products that will help in the elimination of fissures. The "Skin Care" section (see page 143) also has a list of products that keep your skin soft and callus free—thus preventing fissures.

Plantar Warts

Plantar warts occasionally rear their ugly heads on the sole of the foot (the *plantar* surface) and cause foot pain. They can appear and then disappear suddenly, without any effort on your part, and may not recur for years. Usually painful from the pressure of standing and walking, plantar warts

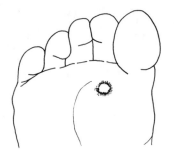

Plantar wart

can become more painful due to sports activities. These warts are typically small, hard, granulated lumps on the skin that can be flesh-colored, white, pink, brown, or gray. They can also feel spongy, thick, and scaly. You may feel as though you have a small stone in your shoe when a wart appears.

Plantar warts are benign tumors caused by common viral infections, usually the human papillomavirus. They generally enter the sole of the foot through cuts and breaks in the skin. The period of time between contact and the wart making its presence known may be several months. There are three types of plantar warts. The first is a single, isolated wart. The second is one wart, often called the "mother," surrounded by any number of smaller "daughter" warts. The third type is a cluster of many warts grouped together, usually on the heels or the balls of the feet. Plantar warts are irregular in shape. While usually small on the skin's surface, they penetrate deep into the foot, where they can cause deep pain.

Moist, cracked skin and open or healing blisters leave one susceptible to the virus. To avoid getting a virus, do not walk barefoot in communal showers or bathrooms. Use thongs, shower booties, or even your shoes or boots. Plantar warts thrive in the warm, moist environment found in sports shoes, so be sure to air your feet when able and change into fresh shoes and socks after participating in sports.

Treating Plantar Warts

Most warts disappear without treatment in four to five months. Sometimes though, when the wart is bothersome or has not gone away on its own, treatment is necessary. While there are over-the-counter plantar-wart removal compounds available, care must be taken in their use. Many products contain salicylic acid. Follow the product's directions to avoid damaging good tissue. Usually the treatment consists of applying the medication and covering the area with a bandage—repeating daily until the problem is resolved. Check your local drugstore or pharmacy for a complete line of

Duct Tape for Wart Removal?

A study reported in the *Archives of Pediatrics and Adolescent Medicine*[29] identified duct tape, the all-purpose household fix-it with hundreds of uses, as an effective wart remover. Researchers say over-the-hardware-counter duct tape is a more effective, less painful alternative to liquid nitrogen, which is used to freeze warts. In the study, patients wore duct tape over their warts for six days. Then they removed the tape, soaked the area in water, and used an emery board or pumice stone to scrape the spot. The tape was reapplied the next morning. The treatment continued for a maximum of two months or until the wart went away. If you have stubborn warts, this duct tape treatment may be worth a try.

The duct tape irritated the warts, and that apparently caused an immune system reaction that attacked the growths, said researcher Dr. Dean "Rick" Focht III of Cincinnati Children's Hospital Medical Center. He said researchers did not test other kinds of tape, and so they cannot say whether there is anything special about the gray, heavy-duty, fabric-backed tape.

The study was conducted at the Madigan Army Medical Center near Tacoma, Wash. It began with 61 patients between the ages of 3 and 22, but only 51 patients completed the study. Of the 26 patients treated with duct tape, 85 percent got rid of their warts compared with 60 percent of the 25 patients who received the freezing treatment.

Pediatric dermatologist Dr. Anthony J. Mancini of Children's Memorial Hospital in Chicago said he uses a form of duct-tape therapy for warts. He combines duct tape with a topical, over-the-counter wart remover for nightly treatments. "The whole point of this is a nonpainful approach," said Mancini, who was not involved in the study.

products. These include Compound W Wart Remover Gel and Liquid, Dr. Scholl's Clear Away Plantar Salicylic Acid Wart Remover System for Feet, DuoFilm Wart Remover, Wartner Wart Removal System, and Wart-Off Wart Removal. Do not use these products if you are a diabetic. Some individuals report success simply covering the wart with a piece of adhesive tape or even duct tape until the wart falls off. You can use moleskin with a hole cut out to relieve painful pressure on the wart. Most drugstores or pharmacies have a selection of pads with cutouts for this purpose.

The treatments may put sports activities on hold until after the spot heals, generally in about a week. The common medical treatment by podiatrists for plantar warts involves the use of liquid nitrogen to freeze off the wart. Other treatment options include electrical burning, minor surgery, or laser surgery. Check with your podiatrist to determine your treatment options.

Rashes

Capillaritis is a common rash that affects the legs of athletes. Presenting as a "funky" rash, it simply seems to come out of nowhere and without any related injury. The rash is a harmless skin condition in which there are reddish-brown patches caused by leaky capillaries. As the capillaries become inflammed, tiny red dots appear on the skin. The dots form into a flat red patch, which becomes brown and then slowly starts to fade away. Its cause is unknown, but it tends to develop after exercise. Many times the rash will appear under the socks and gaiters. It could be a heat rash from the combination of trapped sweat and hot temperatures. In extreme cases it will present with fluid-filled blisters. It can reoccur and even persist for years.

Prickly heat rash is caused by a blockage of sweat glands in areas of heavy sweating, usually beneath clothing. This rash appears as red, itchy, inflamed bumps.

Other possible rashes include poison oak or poison ivy, or rashes that develop because of sensitivity to soap, lotion, or fabrics. These can be ruled out by a physician if they persist.

Treating Rashes

Capillaritis will disappear on its own over a few weeks. The use of a hydro-cortisone 1 percent cream will help control the rash and any related itching. A dermatologist or general physician can be consulted if it does not go away on its own.

Prickly heat rash usually lasts for a few days and then disappears on its own, although it may last longer if hot and humid conditions continue.

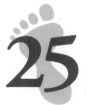

Cold & Heat Therapy

Injuries can be helped through the use of cold and heat therapy. Each has its place in the rehabilitation phase of an injury as they help healing by reducing swelling, reducing pain, and promoting circulation. The rule of thumb is to start with cold and switch to heat or a cold/heat combination later.

Do not use cold or heat therapy on an area where the skin is broken. First treat the wound. Individuals with known or suspected circulatory problems or cold hypersensitivity, paralysis, areas of impaired sensation, or rheumatoid conditions should consult a physician before using cold compression therapy.

Cold Therapy

Cold therapy, sometimes referred to as cryotherapy, is an essential part of rehabilitation after an injury, as well as a prevention measure to avoid problems. Icing is usually done in combination with all the other RICE components: rest, compression, and elevation. Remember that all four are important and should be used together for faster recovery from an injury. Cold therapy can be used for sprains and strains, contusions and bruises, muscle pulls, and post-exercise soreness. Those with Raynaud's syndrome or former frostbite sufferers should not use ice on affected body parts.

Icing progresses through four stages—cold, burning, aching, and finally numbness—usually taking about 20 minutes in all. The numbness stage should be reached in order to receive the full benefits of icing; when the area goes numb, stop applying ice. The duration of icing depends on the type and depth of the injury. Body areas with less fat and tissue should be iced for less time than fatty or dense areas (for example, a bony area less than a hamstring). After an injury, soft-tissue damage can cause uncontrolled swelling. This swelling can increase the damage of the initial injury and increase the healing time. The immediate use of ice will reduce the amount of swelling, tissue damage, blood-clot formation, muscle spasms, inflammation, and pain.

Cold therapy works by decreasing the tissue's temperature and constricting the blood vessels in the injured area. This decreases blood flow, venous/lymphatic drainage, and cell metabolism, reducing the chance of hemorrhage and cell death in an acute injury. Once the fourth stage of icing, numbness, is reached, light range-of-motion can be started. Avoid strenuous exercise during cold therapy.

Cheap Freeze

Homemade ice packs can be made with three parts water and one part rubbing alcohol. Mix in a freezer-grade zip-top bag, and keep one or two in the freezer. The result is a hard slush. If the mix is too hard, let it melt and add a little more alcohol. If it is too liquid, add a little more water. The right consistency will allow the bag to be formed around your foot, ankle, or other body part. Use a towel between the ice bag and your skin. Care must be taken not to get an ice burn from these packs since the alcohol can make them colder than over the counter packs.

Do not place ice directly on the skin. Always use a thin towel, washcloth, or T-shirt between the ice bag and skin. If you have an Ace wrap on the injured part, apply the ice directly over the wrap. Ice cubes in a plastic bag will work, but crushed ice conforms better to the body. When at home use a bag of frozen peas or corn, which conforms nicely to the curves of the foot or ankle. Use an Ace wrap or other type compression wrap to hold the ice against the injured area.

There are two main schools of thought with regard to how long and how frequently to use ice:

- The more typical recommendation is to apply ice three to four times daily to the injured area for 15 to 20 minutes at a time.

- The other recommendation is to ice for 20 minutes, wait 10 minutes, and then reapply the ice for another 20 minutes. Repeat this three times a day for three days after an injury.

TIP:The Ice Masseur Cometh

Ice massage can be done by freezing water in a paper, foam, or plastic cup. When water has frozen, remove part of the cup and rub the ice around the injured area. Because it cools the area faster than normal icing, limit the massage to six to eight minutes at a time, usually three to four times a day. Ice massage is effective when used with range-of-motion exercises and stretching.

Heat Therapy

Heat therapy is used less often than cold therapy. Heat therapy is recommended only after swelling and inflammation have subsided (usually at 48 to 72 hours after an injury). The heat increases blood flow to the injured area, allowing the blood's nutrients to help in the healing process, aid in the removal of waste products from the injured site, and promote healing. Heat can help reduce muscle spasms and pain. Stiffness decreases as tissue elasticity increases. Heat should not be applied for longer than 15 to 20 minutes at a time and should not be applied to areas of broken skin.

Combination Cold & Heat Therapy

A combination of cold and heat therapy can be used 48 to 72 hours after an injury. This can be easily accomplished by alternating the use of cold and heat packs, 10 minutes at a time. An alternative is a contrast bath. Fill two buckets or basins, one with cold water and some ice and the other with tolerable hot water. Alternate your soaking in each for two minutes. With combination therapy, the cold keeps the swelling down while the heat keeps the blood and its nutrients circulating through the injured area.

Dave Barrows, an experienced marathon runner, developed a serious case of bilateral tendinitis. A sports medicine doctor recommended a regimen of contrast baths. Dave had success by following the recommendation:

> Once or twice per day I followed a routine of soaking five minutes at a time for 30 minutes per session, first in an ice bath, then immediately into a 105-degree hot bath, and back and forth five minutes at a time until I had done 15 minutes in each per session. I used a plastic tub for the cold with 10 pounds of crushed ice and water (anything less melts too much before you get to the end of the session). For the hot I filled the bathtub or if at the gym I used the hot tub, which is kept at 104 degrees. I bought a thermometer for checking the temperature of the hot bath at home. Also, a stopwatch is important to keep you honest about the time. As you might expect, this contrast bath surges blood in and out of the feet with good results. It's time consuming but well worth it. Twice a day for 10 days resulted in remarkable improvement for my very serious case.

There are many cold and heat packs available. The list below includes options proven to work well for athletes. Along with cold and heat packs are the many topical creams and gels. Products like Biofreeze (**www.biofreeze .com**), Icyhot (**www.chattem.com**), and Flex-Power Sports Cream (**www .flex-power.com**) can be used for localized muscle pain. Check out your local sports store, drugstore, or pharmacy for more options.

COLD & HEAT PRODUCTS

ACTIVEWRAPS provide heat and cold compression therapy to specific areas of the foot and ankle. It is specifically designed and patented for the unique curvatures of these areas. Each ActiveWrap system includes a comfortable plush medical compression wrap and three hot/cold packs that can be assembled in any position within the wrap. The pack wraps around the foot and stays soft and flexible when cold so they mold comfortably in place. **ActiveWrap, (866) 880-9777, www.activewrap.com**

The **COLD FLEXWRAP** is an all-purpose cold therapy wrap that contours to the foot and ankle as well and other parts of the body: knee, hamstring, neck, shoulder, lower back, and so on. This unique wrap uses a nontoxic gel formulation that never freezes solid; it stays soft and flexible while cold, retaining its therapeutic temperatures for 30 to 40 minutes. It has a soft, velvety fabric covering that eliminates the need to use a towel between the pack and the skin, and protects against ice burn. Elastic straps with Velcro are used to hold the wrap snuggly in place over the injured body part. **Contour Pak, (800) 926-2228, www.contourpak.com**

CRYO-MAX REUSABLE COLD PACKS contain Cryo-Max fluid-filled modules that remain cold for eight hours. The packs can be found in your local drugstores or pharmacies. **Modular Thermal Technologies, (410) 461-4614, www.modularthermaltech.com**

The bandagelike **LIQUID ICE WRAP** is presoaked in the proprietary Liquid Ice solution, which turns cold when removed from its foil package and stays

COLD & HEAT PRODUCTS

cold for up to two hours. You can even apply it and continue playing. Wit the Liquid Ice Recharger and Recovery Pak, you can mix your own Liquid Ice to reuse the bandages. Just add water; soak the dry, rerolled bandage in mix; wring out; and use again or store in an airtight bag. **Americool, (603) 267-7117, www.liquidice.biz**

The **MCDAVID ICE BAG WRAP** provides the ability to use ice and compression simultaneously. The ice bag is enclosed in an adjustable neoprene wrap. **McDavid, (800) 237-8254, www.mcdavidinc.com**

SOLAR POLAR HOT/COLD THERAPY PACKS are hot and cold packs with a unique cross-linked polymer gel that stays soft and pliable even below freezing. Heat and cold is retained for hours. A contoured Ankle Pack is available that uses elastic and Velcro straps to allow a snug fit. Other sizes are offered. Store it in the freezer or place it in the microwave to use as a heat pack. **Thermal Logic, (318) 556-1151, www.thermal-logic.com**

THERMACARE AIR-ACTIVATED HEATWRAPS are made of comfortable, wearable clothlike material that conforms to your body's shape to provide therapeutic heat. Each wrap contains small discs made of natural ingredients that heat up when exposed to air, providing at least eight hours of low-level therapeutic heat on the site of pain. Various sizes are available. Look for these wraps in your drugstore or pharmacy. ThermaCare wraps are made by Proctor & Gamble.

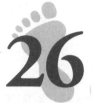

Foot-Care Kits

Consider making three types of foot-care kits. The first is a basic self-care kit for keeping your feet healthy at home. The second is to carry with you in the field or wherever your sport takes you. The third is an event kit for long-distance or multiday activities. Each is equally important.

You can make your own blister kit or purchase a general first-aid kit or a blister medical kit. Most general first-aid kits contain items for basic first-aid care and can be used for blister care by adding a few more specific items. The kits mentioned in the product section below are made specifically for blister care. No matter what each kit contains, you should customize the kit to suit your needs and stock it with sufficient equipment for your outing.

Just the Facts on Foot Care

If you are interested in a pocket-size resource that can be tossed into a gear bag and will supplement these kits, the succinct *Foot Care Field Manual* incorporates many of the treatment ideas from this book. It focuses on helping athletes, crews, and medical support teams know what to do to get themselves or their athlete back onto the course or into the game. Information on this pocket-size manual can be found at **www.fixingyourfeet.com**.

Basic Self-Care Kit

A basic self-care kit for good foot treatment does not have to be large. The following items are recommended; add to the kit as necessary for your particular foot conditions:

☐ Toenail clippers for trimming nails

☐ File or emery board for smoothing nails after clipping

☐ Foot powder for absorbing moisture

☐ Moisturizer cream for softening dry skin, calluses, and corns

☐ Pumice stone for removing calluses and dead skin

☐ Antiseptic ointment for treating cuts and scrapes

Fanny-Pack Kit

If you are an athlete who finds yourself continuously bothered by foot problems, or who often covers long distances without crew support, consider making a small foot-care kit to carry in a fanny pack. Hikers should carry a kit, as part of a larger overall first-aid kit, because of their remoteness from assistance. The following items are recommended:

☐ Tincture of benzoin swabsticks or squeeze vials

☐ Alcohol wipe packets

☐ A fingernail clipper or pin, and matches for blister puncturing

☐ Foot powder in a 35mm film canister (with a salt shaker top; available at backpacking stores)

☐ A small container for your choice of a lubricant

☐ Your choice of tapes wrapped around a pencil

☐ A plastic bag with your choice of blister materials and several pieces of toilet paper or tissues

☐ A small pocket knife with a built-in scissors

Depending on your personal needs, you might adding consider a lightweight ankle support; pads for metatarsal, arch, or heel pain; and a heel cup.

Event Kit

If you participate in events in which you or your crew will be providing foot care, a larger kit is necessary. The kit should contain material based on the length and type of event. Do not rely on medical personnel or aid stations to have the materials you need. The following materials form the core of the kit. Add or eliminate materials based on your personal preferences and experience. Look in the tool section of your local hardware stores for a plastic tool box with trays in which to store the materials.

- ☐ Lubricant of choice
- ☐ Powder of choice
- ☐ Blister patches of choice in various sizes
- ☐ 2nd Skin in various sizes
- ☐ Tapes of choice in a variety of sizes
- ☐ Tincture of benzoin or other tape adherent
- ☐ Swabs for applying benzoin
- ☐ Alcohol pads
- ☐ One DuoDerm pad
- ☐ Tube of 2 percent Xylocaine jelly
- ☐ Gauze pads (2 inch by 2 inch and 4 by 4) for draining blisters
- ☐ Toenail clippers
- ☐ Nail or pedicure file
- ☐ Sharp-pointed scissors
- ☐ Utility scissors for cutting tape

- ☐ Tweezers for pulling blister skin to cut a hole in it
- ☐ Shoehorn
- ☐ Betadine for cleaning dirty wounds/blisters
- ☐ Antiseptic ointment
- ☐ Hydrogen peroxide
- ☐ Extra socks
- ☐ Self-adhering wrap
- ☐ Ace wrap
- ☐ Ankle support
- ☐ Pads for metatarsal, arch, or heel pain
- ☐ Latex gloves
- ☐ Antibacterial hand wipes
- ☐ Small basin for soaking feet
- ☐ Sponge for cleaning feet
- ☐ Hand towel for drying feet
- ☐ Plastic bags for garbage

FOOT-CARE KIT PRODUCTS

BRAVE SOLDIER ANTISEPTIC HEALING OINTMENT was made for athletes and is popular among bicyclists. Developed by a dermatologist as an effective treatment to keep abrasion wounds moist and protected, Brave Soldier helps heal blisters, road rash, minor cuts, and burns. It's made with tea tree oil as a natural antiseptic, aloe gel for its natural healing properties, jojoba oil as a natural moisturizer, vitamin E for rebuilding collagen and skin tissue, shark liver oil for reducing scarring, and comfrey for stimulating skin-cell growth and wound resurfacing. **Brave Soldier, (888) 711-BRAVE, www.bravesoldier.com**

The **SOLO MEDICAL KIT** contains moleskin, tape, tincture of benzoin, and a broad selection of bandaging materials. The kit comes in a zippered nylon pouch. **Outdoor Research, (888) 4OR-GEAR, www.orgear.com**

SPENCO'S BLISTER KIT contains six 2nd Skin 1-inch squares, six sheets of Adhesive Knit, and one sheet of Pressure Pad ovals. The kit comes in a resealable pouch. Look for this kit in backpacking or sporting goods stores. **Spenco Medical Corporation, (800) 877-3626, www.spenco.com**

SUPER SALVE is an antioxidant, antibacterial, and antifungal salve that helps soothe and heal dry and cracked skin, abrasions, and skin conditions common to harsh environments. It's made with a combination of herbs including chaparral leaf, echinacea flower, hops flower, and usnea moss. **Super Salve, (505) 539-2768, www.supersalve.com**

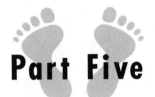

Part Five

Sources & Resources

Appendix A: Product Sources

Rather than use this book as a definitive source for products, use it as a guide to the wide variety of foot-care products available. New products are always being developed. Remember, too, your local stores are an excellent source for what is current in the foot-care marketplace.

When products are mentioned in the text, the company name, telephone number, and Website (if available) are provided. Generally, your first source for most of these products should be your local stores. Ask at your sporting goods store, running store, backpacking or camping store, pharmacy or drugstore, medical supply store, or orthopedic supply store for the products mentioned. While they may not stock all the products, they may be willing to place a special order. Please be aware that not all companies listed in this book sell retail and therefore their products may have to be ordered through a retailer or medical professional. Please respect their sales policies.

The following companies are sources of many of the products listed in this book:

FOOTSMART, (800) 870-7149, **www.footsmart.com**. Sells online and through a print catalogue. They carry a wide assortment of products for flat feet, arch problems, plantar fasciitis, Achilles tendinitis, toenails, bunions, hammertoes, corns, calluses, and skin disorders.

MEDCO SPORTS MEDICINE, (800) 556-3326, **www.medco-athletics.com**. Sells online and through a print catalogue. Products include tapes; self-adhering wraps; tape adherents and skin tougheners; various grades of moleskin; lubricants; powders; antifungal sprays and powders; first-aid equipment; alcohol and tincture of benzoin prep pads; hot and cold therapy equipment; physical therapy equipment; ankle supports; Achilles tendon and plantar fasciitis straps; insoles and heel cups; most Cramer, Mueller, and Spenco products; and Johnson & Johnson Band-Aid Blister Relief, Corn Relief, and Callus Relief.

ZOMBIERUNNER (**www.zombierunner.com**) is a U.S. Internet-based company run by ultrarunners that provides equipment and supplies for trail runners, ultrarunners, and other outdoor enthusiasts. They stock hard to find items like tapes, tape adherents, blister patches, lubricants, powders, gaiters, electrolyte caps, and so on. They specialize in materials prepackaged in foot-care kits.

Appendix D lists medical specialists and companies that often offer products related to their services and business. Check them out for additional options for many of the foot problems and disorders in this book.

You may find products similar to those mentioned which are only available in your area. Watching other athletes and their foot-care habits will often alert you to new products they have found to be useful. Do not hesitate to ask questions when you see new products.

Appendix B:
Shoe & Gear Reviews

Magazines, Websites, and newsletters offer formal reviews of shoes and foot-related gear. The *Fixing Your Feet E-zine,* a free monthly email newsletter, has reviews and information about new foot-care products. The newsletter can be subscribed to at **www.fixingyourfeet.com.**

The print magazines listed below often have additional content on their Websites. Check out their magazine and Website to see the extent of their coverage. Many also post their editorial calendars online, allowing you to see which issues cover shoes and boots.

Adventure Sports **Magazine**
PO Box 926
Grayson, GA 30017
(770) 277-9440
www.adventuresportsmagazine.com

Backpacker **Magazine**
Rodale Press, Inc.
33 E. Minor St.
Emmaus, PA 18098
(800) 666-3434
www.bpbasecamp.com
Annual Gear Guide in March; frequent shoe and boot reviews other months.

Hooked on the Outdoors **Magazine**
11 Dunwoody Park, Suite 140
Atlanta, GA 30338
(770) 396-4320

www.ruhooked.com
Occasional footwear reviews.

Inside Triathlon **Magazine**
1830 N. 55th St.
Boulder, CO 80301-2703
(303) 440-0601
www.insidetriathlon.com

Marathon & Beyond **Magazine**
411 Park Lane Dr.
Champaign, IL 61820
(217) 359-9345
www.marathonandbeyond.com
Occasional articles on sports injuries and fitness.

Outside Magazine
400 Market St.
Santa Fe, NM 87501
(800) 678-1131
www.outsidemag.com
The Buyer's Guide is a special
magazine typically issued in May.

Runner's World Magazine
Rodale Press, Inc.
33 E. Minor St. Emmaus, PA
18098
(800) 666-2828
www.runnersworld.com
The April (spring), and October
(fall), and December (winter)
issues usually have shoe reviews.

Running Times Magazine
213 Danbury Rd.
Wilton, CT 06897
(203) 761-1113
www.runningtimes.com
The March (spring) and
September (fall) issues usually
have shoe reviews.

Trail Runner Magazine
1101 Village Rd., UL-4D
Carbondale, CO 81623
(970) 704-1442
www.trailrunnermag.com
The spring and fall issues usually
have shoe reviews.

Triathlete Magazine
328 Encinitas Blvd., Suite 100
Encinitas, CA 92024
(760) 634-4100
www.triathletemag.com

UltraRunning Magazine
PO Box 890238
Weymouth, MA 02189-0238
(781) 340-0616
www.ultrarunning.com
Occasional gear reviews and articles
with personal experiences and tips.

Appendix C:
Medical & Footwear Specialists

American Academy of Orthopaedic Surgeons
6300 N. River Rd.
Rosemont, IL 60018-4262
(800) 346-AAOS
www.aaos.org

American Academy of Podiatric Sports Medicine
PO Box 723
Rockville, MD 20848-0723
(888) 854-3388
www.aapsm.org

American Chiropractors Association
1701 Clarendon Blvd.
Arlington, VA 22209
(800) 986-4636
www.americhiro.org

American Massage Therapy Association
820 Davis St., Suite 100
Evanston, IL 60201-4444
(847) 864-0123
www.amtamassage.org

American Orthopaedic Foot and Ankle Society
2517 Eastlake Ave. East, Suite 200
Seattle, WA 98102
(800) 235-4855
www.aofas.org

American Orthotics and Prosthetics Association
330 John Carlyle St., Suite 200
Alexandria, VA 22314
(571) 431-0876
www.aopanet.org

American Physical Therapy Association
1111 N. Fairfax St.
Alexandria, VA 22314-1488
(800) 999-2782
www.apta.org

American Podiatric Medical Association
9312 Old Georgetown Rd.
Bethesda, MD 20814-1698
(800) FOOTCARE
www.apma.org

International Chiropractic Association
1110 N. Glebe Rd. #1000
Arlington, VA 22201
(800) 423-4690
www.chiropractic.org

National Athletic Trainers' Association
2952 Stemmons Freeway
Dallas, TX 75247
(214) 637-6282
www.nata.org

Pedorthic Footwear Association
7150 Columbia Gateway Dr., Suite G
Columbia, MD 21046
(410) 381-7278
www.pedorthics.org

Appendix D:
Feet-Related Websites

A free monthly email newsletter of the same name as this book is offered at **www.fixingyourfeet.com.** The e-zine contains articles on feet-related issues and helps athletes learn about new foot-care techniques and products between editions of the book. Old issues are archived at the site.

About Walking
www.walking.about.com

The Active Foot & Ankle Care Center
www.drrun.com

The Ambulatory Foot Clinic—Podiatric Pain Management Center
www.footcare4u.com

Center for Sports Medicine & Orthopaedics
www.sportmed.com

Dr. Pribut's Running Injuries Page
www.drpribut.com/sports/
sportframe.html

Eneslow Foot Comfort Center
www.eneslow.com

Feet Fixer.com
www.feetfixer.com

Foot and Ankle Link Library
www.footandankle.com/podmed

Footcare Direct—Target In on Your Foot Care Solutions
www.footcaredirect.com

Foot Express—Footcare Home Health Products & Treatments
www.footexpress.com

The Foot Health Network
www.foot.com

The Foot Store—Specializing in Foot and Heel Pain Treatment
www.footstore.com

Foot Web—Footcare Treatment Information Resource
www.footweb.com

My Foot Shop—Your Source for Healthy Feet
www.myfootshop.com

Our Foot Doctor.com
www.ourfootdoctor.com

Running Barefoot
www.runningbarefoot.org

Society for Barefoot Living
www.barefooters.org

Support Your Feet
www.supportyourfeet.com/
index.html

Notes

1 Roland Mueser, *Long-Distance Hiking: Lessons from the Appalachian Trail* (Camden, ME: Rugged Mountain Press, 1998), p. 32.

2 J. J. Knapik, K. I. Reynolds, K. L. Duplantis, and B. H. Jones, "Friction Blisters: Pathophysiology, Prevention and Treatment," *Sports Medicine* 20, no. 3 (1995), p. 140.

3 Karen Berger, *Advanced Backpacking* (New York: W. W. Norton & Company, 1998), pp. 69–70.

4 The usual issues are *Backpacking* (March, the Annual Gear Guide Issue), *Outside* (May Buyer's Guide), *Runner's World* (April and September), *Running Times* (March and September), and *Trail Runner* (spring and fall).

5 J. D. Denton, Dennis Grandy, DPM, and Tom Kennedy, "How to Find the Right Shoe for You," *Running Times* (September 1996), p. 16, and "How to Find a Shoe That Works," *Running Times* (March 1997), p. 18.

6 Tom Brunick and Bob Wischnia, "Choosing the Right Shoe" and "Know Your Foot Type," *Runner's World* (April 1997), p. 52.

7 J. J. Knapik, K. L. Reynolds, K. L. Duplantis, and B. H. Jones, "Friction Blisters: Pathophysiology, Prevention, and Treatment," *Sports Medicine* 20, no. 3 (1995), p. 142.

8 12 miles per day times, 5,280 feet/mile divided by 2.5 feet/step. For each mile more than 12, add 2100 steps. For each mile less than 12, subtract 2100 steps.

9 Ray Jardine, *The Pacific Crest Trail Hiker's Handbook* (LaPine, OR: Adventure Lore Press, 1996), p. 93.

10 Tim Noakes, MD, *The Lore of Running* (Champaign, IL: Leisure Press, 1991), p. 460.

11 Robert Boeder, *Beyond the Marathon: The Grand Slam of Trail Ultrarunning* (Vienna, GA: Old Mountain Press, 1996), p. 22.

12 J. J. Knapik, K. L. Reynolds, K. L. Duplantis, and B. H. Jones, "Friction Blisters: Pathophysiology, Prevention and Treatment," *Sports Medicine* 20, no. 3 (1995), p. 139.

13 Andrew Lovy, "New Blister Formula Revealed! Free!" *UltraRunning* (April 1990), p. 40.

[14] Richard Benyo, *The Death Valley 300: Near-Death and Resurrection on the World's Toughest Endurance Course* (Forestville: Specific Publications, 1991), p. 142.

[15] Colin Fletcher, *The Complete Walker III* (New York: Alfred A. Knopf, 1996), p. 86.

[16] Gary Cantrell, "From the South: The Amazing Miracle of Duct Tape," *UltraRunning* (December, 1988), pp. 36–37.

[17] Donald Baxter, MD; David Porter, MD, PhD; Paul Flahavan, C.Ped; and Charles May, "The Ideal Running Orthosis: A Philosophy of Design," *Biomechanics* (March 1996), pp. 41–44.

[18] Tim Noakes, MD, *The Lore of Running* (Champaign, IL: Leisure Press, 1991), p. 459.

[19] J. J. Knapik, K. L. Reynolds, K. L. Duplantis, and B. H. Jones, "Friction Blisters: Pathophysiology, Prevention and Treatment," *Sports Medicine* 20, no. 3 (1995), p. 138.

[20] Ibid, p. 140.

[21] Ibid, p. 139.

[22] Bryan Bergeron, MD, "A Guide to Blister Management," *The Physician and Sportsmedicine* (February 1995), p. 40.

[23] Ibid, p. 43.

[24] William Trolan, MD, *Blister Fighter Guide* (Seattle: Outdoor Research, 1996).

[25] Auleley, Guy-Robert, MD, et al, "Validation of the Ottowa Ankle Rules," *Annals of Emergency Medicine* 32, no. 1 (July 1998), pp. 14–18.

[26] "The Conservative Treatment of Plantar Fasciitis: A Prospective Randomized, Multicenter Outcome Study" (American Orthopaedic Foot and Ankle Society, October 1996).

[27] Robert Nirschl, MD, MS, "Plantar Fasciitis—A New Perspective," *American Medical Joggers Association AMAA Quarterly* (summer 1996).

[28] Karen Maloney Backstrom, C. Forsyth, B. Walden, Abstract: "Comparison of Two Methods of Stretching the Gastrocnemius and Their Effects on Ankle Range of Motion" (University of Colorado Health Services Center, Denver, CO, April 1994).

[29] Dean R. Focht III, MD; Carole Spicer, RN; and Mary P. Fairchok, MD, "The Efficacy of Duct Tape vs Cryotherapy in the Treatment of Verruca Vulgaris (the Common Wart)," *Archives of Pediatric Adolescent Medicine* 156, no. 10 (October 2002).

Glossary

Achilles tendon—the large tendon that runs from the calf to the back of the heel.

adventure racing—multisport races over difficult terrain, often done in teams over several days.

arch—the curved part of the bottom of the foot.

athlete's foot—a fungal infection that causes itchy, red, soggy, flaking, and cracking skin between the toes or fluid-filled bumps on the sides or sole of the foot.

biomechanics—the study of the mechanics of a living body, especially of the forces exerted by muscles and gravity on the skeletal structure.

blister—a fluid-filled sac between layers of skin that occurs as a result of friction.

bone spur—a small, bony growth usually indicating a bone irritation.

bruise—an injury in which blood vessels beneath the skin are broken and blood escapes to produce a discolored area.

bunion—a bony protrusion at the base of the big toe.

bunionette—a bunion on the small toe.

bursitis—the formation of an inflamed fluid-filled sac, usually where muscles or tendons glide over bone.

calcaneus—the large heel bone.

callus—the thickening of skin caused by recurring friction, usually on the sole of the foot, heel, or inner big toe.

claw toes—toes that are contracted down at the middle joint but up at the joint at the ball of the foot.

contusion—a bruising injury that does not involve a break in the skin.

corn—a thickening of the skin, generally on or between the toes, usually caused by friction.

dermis—the sensitive connective tissue layer of the skin located below the epidermis, containing nerve endings, sweat and sebaceous glands, and blood and lymph vessels.

dislocation—a complete displacement of bone from its normal position at the joint surface.

edema—the swelling of body tissues due to excessive fluid.

epidermis—the outer, protective, nonvascular layer of the skin covering the dermis.

eversion—movement of the foot as it rolls inward at the ankle.

fibula—the outer and smaller of the two bones of the lower leg.

fissure—crack in the skin, usually found on the toughened, callused skin of the heels.

flat foot—a foot that has either a low arch or no arch.

forefoot—the ball of the foot and the toes.

frostbite—the result of the freezing of skin tissue.

Haglund's deformity—a bump in the form of an enlargement of the back of the heel bone (calcaneus) at the area of the insertion of the Achilles tendon.

hallux—the great or big toe.

hallux valgus—the turning in of the great toe joint that often causes bunions.

hammertoes—toes that are contracted at the toe's middle joint, making the toe bend upward at its center and forcing the tip of the toe downward.

heel pad—the soft tissue pad on the bottom of the heel.

heel-pain syndrome—pain at the heel usually caused by overuse or repetitive stress to the foot's heel.

heel spur—a small edge of bone that juts out of the calcaneous.

hematoma—a swelling containing blood beneath the skin caused by an injury to a blood vessel.

hot spot—a hot and reddened area of skin that has been irritated by friction.

hyperhidrosis—excessive moisture.

infection—condition in which a part of the body is invaded by a microorganism such as a bacteria or virus.

ingrown toenail—when one or both sides of a toenail that has grown into the flesh of the toe.

inversion—movement of the foot as it rolls outward at the ankle.

last—the form over which a shoe or boot is constructed.

lateral—the outside of the foot, leg, or body.

ligament—the strong, fibrous connective tissue at a joint that connects one bone to another bone.

maceration—a breaking down or softening of skin tissue by extended exposure to moisture.

mallet toes—toes that are contracted at the end joint only.

medial—the inside of the foot, leg, or body.

metatarsal—one of the five bones at the ball of the foot.

metatarsalgia—pain somewhere underneath the metatarsal heads of the foot.

midfoot—the mid or center part of the foot, containing the arch and five metatarsal bones.

Morton's neuroma—pain on the bottom of the foot, usually under the pad of the third or fourth toe.

Morton's toe—a foot type where the second toe is longer than the big toe.

neuroma—the swelling of a nerve due to an inflammation of the nerve or the tissue surrounding the nerve.

NSAIDS—acronym for nonsteroidal anti-inflammatory drugs; used to control pain and swelling after an injury.

orthopedist—an orthopedic surgeon specializing in the treatment and surgery of bones and joint injuries, diseases, and problems.

orthotic—an insert made from a mold of the bottom of the foot that is then inserted into a shoe or boot to correct a foot abnormality.

pedorthist—a specialist trained to work on the fit or modification of shoes and orthotics to alleviate foot problems caused by disease, overuse, or injury.

peripheral neuropathy—a painful nerve condition that can manifest itself as a burning sensation in the feet.

plantar—the bottom surface of the foot.

plantar fascia—the band of fibers along the arch of the foot that connects the heel to the toes.

plantar fasciitis—an inflammation of the plantar fascia.

plantar warts—small, hard, flesh-colored, white, or pink granulated lumps typically found on the feet and caused by a virus.

podiatrist—a doctor of podiatric medicine who specializes in the treatment and surgery of the foot and ankle.

pronation—the rolling of the foot toward the inside of the body when weight bearing.

Raynaud's syndrome—discomfort caused by a decreased blood supply to the fingers and toes.

RICE—acronym for rest, ice, compression, and elevation; describes the typical treatment of sprain and strain injuries.

sesamoiditis—an inflammation of the two little bones beneath the ball of the foot and under the joint that moves the big toe.

sole—the bottom of the foot.

sprain—a joint injury in which ligament damage is sustained.

sterilization—the process by which bacteria is removed.

strain—muscular injury produced by overuse or abuse of a muscle.

stress fracture—typically a small crack in the outer shell of the affected bone caused by sudden or repetitive stress, usually from overuse without proper conditioning.

subluxation—an incomplete or partial dislocation.

subungal hematoma—a hematoma under the nail plate.

supination—the rolling of the foot toward the outside of the body when weight bearing.

tendinitis—an inflammation of a tendon or its surrounding sheath.

tendon—the elastic tough fibrous tissue that connects muscles to bone.

toe box—the front part of a shoe or boot that covers the toes.

toenail fungus—nails that are thick and deformed, with a brown, white, or yellowish discoloration.

transient parasthesia—a temporary nerve compression that can be caused by a gradual buildup of fluids in your feet during extended on-your-feet activity.

trench foot—a serious nonfreezing cold injury that develops when the skin of the feet is exposed to a combination of moisture and cold for extended periods.

turf toe—a condition of pain at the base of the big toe at the ball of the foot, usually caused from jamming the toe.

ultrarunning—running distances greater than a marathon.

virus—a tiny organism that causes disease.

wart—a thickened, painful area of skin caused by a virus.

Bibliography

Copeland, Glen. *The Foot Book: Relief for Overused, Abused & Ailing Feet.* John Wiley & Sons, 1992.

Ellis, Joe, DPM, with Joe Henderson. *Running Injury-Free.* Emmaus, PA: Rodale Press, 1994.

Jardine, Ray. *The Pacific Crest Trail Hiker's Handbook.* LaPine, OR: Adventure Lore Press, 1996 (out of print).

Levine, Suzanne M., MD. *My Feet Are Killing Me!* New York: McGraw-Hill Book Company, 1987 (out of print).

McGann, Daniel M., DPM, and L. R. Robinson. *The Doctor's Sore Foot Book.* New York: William Morrow and Company, Inc., 1991 (out of print).

Noakes, Tim, MD. *The Lore of Running.* Human Kinetics, 4th ed., 2003.

Salmans, Sandra. *Your Feet: Questions You Have...Answers You Need.* Allentown, PA: People's Medical Society, 1998 (out of print).

Schneider, Myles J., DPM, and Mark D. Sussman, DPM. *How to Doctor Your Feet Without a Doctor.* Washington, DC: Acropolis Books, Ltd., 1984 (out of print).

Subotnick, Steven I., DPM, MS. *The Running Foot Doctor.* San Francisco: World Publications, 1977 (out of print).

——, *Sports & Exercise Injuries: Conventional, Homeopathic & Alternative Treatments.* Berkeley, CA: North Atlantic Books, 1991.

Taliaferro Blauvelt, Carolyn, and Nelson, Fred R. T. *A Manual of Orthopaedic Terminology,* 6th ed. St. Louis: Mosby, 1998.

Tremain, David M., MD, and Awad, Elias M., PhD. *The Foot & Ankle Sourcebook.* McGraw-Hill/Contemporary Books; 2nd ed., 1998.

Trolan, William, MD. *Blister Fighter Guide.* Seattle: Outdoor Research, 1996.

Weisenfeld, Murry F., MD, with Barbara Burr. *The Runner's Repair Manual.* New York: St. Martin's Press, 1980 (out of print).

About the Author

John Vonhof brings a varied background and extensive experience to *Fixing Your Feet*. This third edition, which he wrote and illustrated, is the synthesis of over 26 years of experience as a runner and hiker.

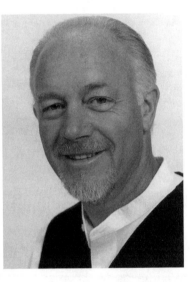

In between editions of *Fixing Your Feet*, John's free monthly email newsletter, *Fixing Your Feet E-zine*, serves to inform and educate athletes about all that's new in foot care. His *Foot Care Manual* helps athletes, coaches, trainers, support crews, and medical staffs fix problems out in the field, where sports happen. Both these publications are described at **www.fixing yourfeet.com**.

A runner since 1982, John discovered trail running and ultras in 1984. He has completed more than 20 ultras: 50K's 50-milers, 100-milers, 24-hour runs, and a 72-hour run. He completed the difficult Western States 100-mile Endurance Run three times and the Santa Rosa 24-Hour and 12-Hour Track Runs 12 times. In 1987, with fellow runner Will Uher, John fastpacked the 211-mile John Muir Trail in the Sierra Nevada in 8½ days, carrying a 30-pound pack.

As the Ohlone Wilderness 50K Trail Run race director for 15 years, John worked at providing a quality event for runners of all skill levels who participated in this arduous trail ultra.

In 1992 John changed careers, becoming a paramedic, orthopedic technician, and emergency-room technician. He now works for an emergency medical services agency in the San Francisco Bay Area as a prehospital care coordinator.

Over the years John has provided volunteer medical aid at numerous sporting events, patching feet and providing advice to thousands of athletes. He continues to be sought out for his expertise and experience in providing answers to foot-care questions.

General Index

Product Index